Special Women

The Role of the Professional Labor Assistant

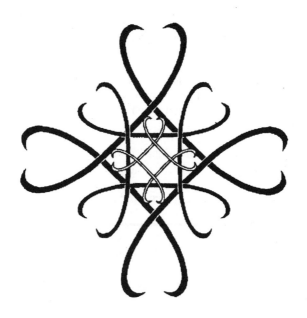

Paulina Perez
&
Cheryl Snedeker

Cutting Edge Press

P9-DVI-881

The symbol you see on the inside cover page, and throughout the book, is a variation of the hooked diamond pattern, which appears in traditional rugs, textiles and wall hangings made by women in cultures all over the world. The sign of the hooked diamond is a birth symbol, which, according to Sheila Kitzinger, anthropologist and writer on childbirth, "represents both vagina and uterus and is the counterpart of the male phallic symbol. Whereas everyone is aware of phallic symbolism in art, the birth symbol has been largely ignored"
Designers Penny Simkin and Lydia Kinata selected the hooked diamond as the inspiration for these symbols, using several "layers" to create a sense of depth to the diamond, and adding curved lines to suggest the soft contours of the female body.

Cutting Edge Press
A division of Perez Enterpises, Inc
287 Whiteface Mountain Dr.
Johnson, VT 05656

The information contained in this book is not intended as a substitute for consulting with your physician, midwife or other health care provider. Any attempt to diagnose and treat an illness should be done under the direction of a health care professional. The publisher does not advocate the use of any particular health care protocol, but believes that the information in this book should be available to the public. The publisher and author are not responsible for any adverse effects or consequences resulting from the use of any suggestions or procedures discussed in this book. Should the reader have any questions concerning the appropriateness for any procedures mentions, the author and publisher strongly suggest consulting a health care professional.

While the advice and information in this book are believed to be true and accurate at the date of going to press, neither the author nor the publisher can accept any legal responsibility for any errors or omissions that may be made. The publisher makes no warranty, express or implied, with respect to the matter contained therein.

©2000 by Paulina G. Perez

First Edition, May 1990
Second Edition, August 1994
Revised and Updated Third Edition , June 2000
1990, 1994, 2000 by Paulina Perez
All rights reserved
Printed in the United States of America

Book Design and Layout by Cheryl Snedeker
Cover Design by Jim Fitzgerald

Library of Congress Cataloging in Publication Data
Perez, Paulina and Snedeker, Cheryl
Special Women: The Role of the Professional Labor Assistant

Library of Congress Catalog Card Number
94-94211
ISBN
0-9641159-9-9
1. Obstetrics--popular work 2.Childbirth– social aspects 3.
Education–medical I. Title

Part of Chapter 10, "Managing Conflict With Medical Staff (pp. 108-113) is copyrighted by Henci Goer, 1990.

To Cheri -
For her unwavering support for the role of the
professional labor assistant in obstetrics.
--PGP

For Devyn -- whose birth changed my life
--CAS

Contents

Acknowledgments

This book would never have been written without the people who've helped me grow.

Mollie Fern Sumrall Gandy, an incredible woman, who taught me what strength and courage are all about and whose presence is with me constantly. The part I remember most about her is that she could play a mean game of Chinese checkers.

Theda and A.P. Gandy, who taught me that I could do anything I set my mind to, and who smiled and sometimes worried while I did just that.

Eric, who has loved me unconditionally for the last twenty five years, who supports me always, and who wakes to kiss me goodbye at 3am when I leave for a birth.

Bryan, Mark and Scott, whose births taught me much about myself, whose lives have taught me about patience and commitment, and who have put up with a mother who sometimes leaves for days at a time.

Jane Gandy, without whose advocacy in a hospital this revised addition would not have been possible.

All the mothers and babies I've cared for over the years and who have given me a lifetime of memories.

...from Cheryl Snedeker

Mike, whose career has both improved and ruined my life, whose encouragement has kept me strong and sane, and whose love is the only constant in an ever-changing world.

Both Cheryl and I want to thank the many parents and professionals who wrote the articles and birth stories which are included in this book: Douglas Thibodeaux, M.D., Bethany Hays, M.D., Harlan Ellis, M.D., Beth Shearer, Henci Goer, Grace Couch, Heather Mitchell, Lori Sisto, Kathleen Hardy, Juliet Brown, Lynn Badger, Denise Driscoll, Eileen Thibodeaux, Lisa Spracklin, Guadalupe Trueba, Kathy Bradley, Teresa Howard, Lisa Klaehn, Robin Rabenschlag,,Joni Nichols, Robyn Mattox, Crystal Sada, Karen Kilson, Diane Tinker, Teri Gulker, Stephanie Soderblom, Kim Greenlee, Deb Sexton, Sue Frizzell, Connie Banack, Tracey de Hoop, Carol Rotolo, Janice Pearson, and Clive Pohl.

Since the publication of the first edition of *Special Women*, I have been blessed to have been able to educate and communicate with prospective doulas and monitrices throughout North America. I am most appreciative of their willingness to share stories of their accomplishments as well as their frustrations. This has helped add more depth to my educational seminars.

Being able to collaborate with dedicated primary caregivers who welcome labor support for their clients has been useful to both me and to the families I serve. My world has been enriched by being able to work with and learn from Douglas Thibodeaux, M.D., Stephen Guilliams, M.D., Catherine Maxwell-Hees, M.D., Bethany Hays, M.D., Patricia Jones, C.N.M., and Marje Kelso, C.N.M.

Introduction

My own work as a monitrice planted the seed for this book. I could not find much written about this role I had chosen, and I often found myself thinking about how others would handle a given situation. My work as a nurse consultant and public speaker helped the seed germinate. Whenever I lectured, women would approach me with questions about how to set up a practice, how to decide what role to play (monitrice or doula), and how I felt about different aspects of my work. The seed had turned into a seedling by the time I decided to tackle the writing of the book. Because I felt strongly about including information from others as well as from myself, I designed questionnaires to be completed by "those of us in the field," as well as from families who had chosen to hire professional labor support. I surveyed approximately 75 families and 55 professionals. The generalizations in this book are based on those surveys. I have chosen quite often to include in the text the actual words of those surveyed.

As I compiled all the date from the surveys, the seedling became a much stronger plant. The book began to take form. The more I wrote, the more I realized the book needed to be written. The research continued. My publisher, Penny Simkin, continued to urge me to keep cultivating this plant when I sometimes thought this was an endless task. After several years watching this plant grow, I decided that I needed someone to help me prune it, weed around it, and give it more direction. That help came in the form of Cheryl Snedeker. I had first met Cheryl when she hired me as her professional labor assistant. That relationship turned into a friendship and her daughter Devyn is not only one of "my babies" but has become the daughter I never had. Her interest in this book and its subject matter, as well as her talent as a writer made her the perfect choice to help me. We worked well together and *Special Women* had new life. The plant was beginning to blossom.

As I was beginning to think about picking the blossoms to present the bouquet to you -- those who work as labor support professionals and those who want to become labor support professionals -- I became very ill. My family, friends, and the book kept me going. I had to get well; the book had to be finished. Cheryl flew to Houston from her home in Michigan and did most of the computer work while I sat next to her. I slowly recovered and the book was finally finished. The plant has produced blossoms for you to enjoy. As you read this book, realize that the information in it came from some very *Special Women* -- women who have chosen to take on the very difficult, but rewarding work of a monitrice or doula, and the mothers they have cared for.

1.
What is the Professional Labor Assistant?

"My labor assistant was my friend, my strength, my shield, my teacher, and, most of all, my anchor in a sea of confusion, pain and fatigue. She was to me what a lighthouse was to a ship, a gentle guide showing you your destination and helping you avoid unnecessary hazards."   A Mother

"The labor assistant is often the only link from pregnancy to birth to post-partum."   A Monitrice

"I can't believe that obstetricians are resistant to utilizing a labor assistant. She makes labor and delivery so easy physicians should be beating a path to her door."   An Obstetrician

Birth can be a positive and life-changing experience for a woman. It can be a time of great introspection for the mother-to-be as she feels her body working to bring forth new life. It can be a time when she is surrounded by family and friends. A time for wonder and joy. Joanne feels that way about the birth of her daughter. She had planned for this birth carefully. Since her husband traveled frequently, her obstetrician had suggested hiring professional labor support in case Jeff had to be out of town while Joanne was in labor. She found a monitrice and contacted her for a prenatal visit. Both Joanne and Jeff liked Sally and felt secure that she would be there for Joanne if Jeff couldn't be. When labor started, Jeff was at home, but they called the monitrice early in labor for reassurance that everything was going well.

Joanne labored at home, with the support of Sally and Jeff. She walked about, watched a rented movie, ate some toast, and soaked in a warm tub. She felt comfortable with the pains of labor and confident that she would be okay. When she reached seven centimeters dilatation, Sally suggested they make plans to go to the hospital. Joanne called her best friend Jan who was going to meet them there and headed out. When they arrived at the hospital, Joanne was shown to the birthing room, where Jan was already anxiously waiting. Joanne met her hospital obstetrical nurse, who took some readings on the fetal monitor and asked some medical questions.

Joanne's labor progressed slowly but surely. Jeff and Sally walked the corridors of the hospital with her, stopping to rub her back during contractions and to encourage her to relax and let go. When she reached transition, Jeff rubbed her lower back almost constantly, and Sally supplied some much appreciated ice water. When Joanne started to push, she had one arm around her friend Jan and one arm around her husband Jeff. With their support and encouragement she finally gave birth to a healthy little girl. Joanne put her daughter to breast almost immediately and the baby nursed hungrily. Joanne was filled with wonder and awe as she looked at her tiny daughter, and as she looked around the room at the others who were there to share this experience, she felt full of love.

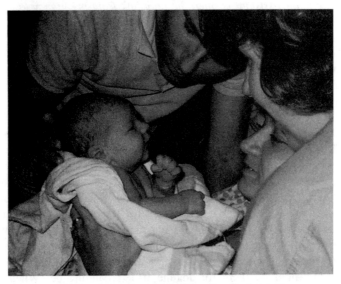

The labor assistant has helped this couple make their birth
a truly unforgettable event.

Joanne's birth experience is the kind of birth that every woman deserves. She was surrounded by people who cared for her and helped her to achieve her goal of a natural birth. And even though it was not an easy birth, Joanne never felt that she needed anesthesia for pain relief. When a contraction seemed particularly hard to deal with and painful, Sally was always there stroking her leg or arm, telling her that she knew it hurt but it would be over soon.

Unfortunately, not all woman receive the kind of support that Joanne had during her birth experience.

Marcia's labor began with erratic contractions and she was excited to know that she'd soon see her baby. After a few hours her contractions where five minutes apart and even though they didn't hurt too much she thought she should be at the hospital. She and her husband Fred arrived at the hospital and were ushered into a beautifully decorated labor-delivery-recovery room. About this time Marcia noted that her contractions didn't seem as strong as they did at home. When the nurse examined her, it was uncomfortable as her cervix was still posterior. The nurse told her she was two centimeters dilated and that it would be quite a while before the baby would be born. Marcia turned to Fred and asked "Do you think we should go home and wait for labor to get stronger?" Fred was worried that he wouldn't know when to bring Marcia back to the hospital and so he said "Why don't we stay a while and see what happens." So Marcia put on a hospital gown and climbed into bed for what she thought was going to be a short time. After all her birth plan said that she wanted to walk during labor.

Blood work was drawn from her arm and two elastic belts were strapped around her abdomen. Fred was intrigued with the tracing from the fetal monitor and watched it constantly. He commented that it had been quite some time since the last contraction. The thought occurred to Marcia that maybe this was false labor, but she pushed it out of her mind. She really wanted it to be labor and surely if this was false labor, she decided the nurses would send her home.

After an hour or so, it really seemed like nothing was happening, so she turned on the TV. As she watched the TV, she realized she was hungry. When she asked Fred to go get her something to eat, the nurse quickly interjected you can't eat or drink anything while you're in labor. When Marcia told the nurse how thirsty she was, the nurse said perhaps Marcia was a little dehydrated and that an IV would help her. Fred nodded in agreement while the nurse began getting her equipment to start the IV. After the IV had been running, Marcia noticed she still felt thirsty.

Marcia was really anxious about what was going on, but since she was already at the hospital, she decided to stay. At about that time, the doctor on call for her physician came in and examined her. He said there had been no change since the nurse's exam several hours earlier, except that her cervix was now anterior. He suggested breaking her bag of waters to speed things up. The nurse immediately handed him what looked like a long crochet hook as Marcia said, "Whatever you think is best."

Shortly after the doctor left, Marcia's contractions got a little stronger. This was a little scary, but it helped that Fred was right by her side reminding her to relax and breathe. Her nurse, Jane, told her what a good job she was doing with her breathing. Marcia and Fred really liked Jane and began to rely on Jane's help a lot. When Jane told them a few hours later, that Marcia's contractions weren't close enough together and that the doctor wanted to start pitocin to help things along, they didn't ask any questions. They felt it would be okay, after all Jane was going to be there to help them. Marcia had now been at the hospital for six hours.

The pitocin worked quickly and Marcia's contractions got closer and stronger. Now Marcia really felt scared and held Fred's hand tightly as she did her rhythmic breathing techniques. She asked Jane, "Do you think I need a little medicine?" Fred wondered about that too. He had never seen Marcia in pain like this before. Jane's reply was, "You're in good control, just focus on Fred when you have a contraction." Hearing that made both Marcia and Fred feel better instantly.

Half an hour later, Jane told Fred and Marcia that her shift was over and that Gayle would be their new nurse. As vulnerable as Marcia felt, she immediately began to worry. As Gayle came on duty she mentioned that it was very busy now with many women in labor. Because of that she would be in and out of the room. Marcia hurt a lot now and was really scared. When Gayle examined her and said you're three centimeters now, Marcia began to panic. She'd been at the hospital over eight hours and was just three centimeters. She felt very dejected and looked up at Fred and said "I can't stand this anymore. I need something for the pain." Gayle told Fred and Marcia not to worry, she'd go get the anesthesiologist to give her an epidural. Marcia said "But I didn't want to have anesthesia." Gayle patted her hand and said most women need anesthesia and that she too had had an epidural during labor. She turned to Fred and said "You don't want to see her suffer any more do you?" Fred quickly responded, "Go get the anesthesiologist."

Within forty five minutes, Marcia felt no pain and she and Fred had the TV on again. They thought everything was going wonderfully until the doctor returned a few hours later and said when he examined her, "You're only four centimeters and the baby is very big. You don't seem to be progressing. We'll give you another hour and if nothing happens we may have to do a cesarean."

This was the first time that Marcia and Fred had thought about a cesarean. Sure, they knew that the cesarean rate was around 30 percent in their hospital, but they had never planned to be in that thirty percent.

Cesareans happened to someone else. They turned to Gayle and asked what to do. Gayle replied, "I'm sure the doctor will do whatever is best."

The hour went by very slowly; Marcia was really frightened. Would this never end? She'd been here over twelve hours now. When the doctor came back, although her cervix she was still four centimeters. He stated "You could go on laboring, but I don't think this is going to work. I think we should go on and do a cesarean before the baby gets in any distress." When Marcia heard the word distress, she immediately said, "I want my baby to be okay, so if you say a cesarean is best..."

An hour later, thirteen hours after she had entered the hospital, Marcia was on the operating table with Fred at her side when the doctor pulled her baby boy into the world. She caught a glimpse of him as they took him to the warmer. After they dried him off, Fred held him next to her for a few minutes before he was taken to the nursery.

When Marcia was taken to the recovery room, she asked Fred to go check on their son. She wanted to nurse him. When Fred left, she really felt alone. And the pain began again, except it was worse than before. The nurse gave her a narcotic for the pain in her IV and she was so groggy that it didn't bother her too much when Fred came back and said the baby had to stay in the nursery because he was a little cold.

Marcia's birth was typical for an American women. She gave birth in the hospital; 99 percent of American woman do. She was cared for by more than one nurse. In fact it is not unusual that she had never met the doctor caring for her during labor. Marcia labored for twelve to thirteen hours, fairly standard for a hospital setting. She reached a point in labor where she couldn't stand the pain any longer and someone suggested an epidural anesthesia. Marcia's nurse was right about women using anesthesia for birth, 60-70 percent of women in the US have some sort of anesthesia during birth. Marcia also joined the ranks of mothers having a cesarean section. Her "failure" to progress made her one of the more than 25 percent of American women who birth by surgery. Following the birth, Marcia's feelings were of joy, relief and surprising to her, emptiness.

Joanne's birth was atypical for a hospital birth in North America. She entered labor prepared, confident, and realistic about the road ahead of her. She labored at home and did not enter the hospital until late in the labor process. She had loving, caring, trusted and trusting people around her who believed in her ability to birth and who helped her work through the pain. Her caregivers safeguarded both her and her infant without making technology the focus of her birth. She birthed without drugs; only one tenth of the American women birthing each year do so. Joanne was awake and aware and able to experience fully one of life's most treasured moments, the birth of her child. After her birth, Joanne felt elated, satisfied and confident.

Contrast the awe-inspiring images of Joanne's birth with the disquieting images of Marcia's delivery. What happened to the birth Marcia wanted? What was different about Joanne's birth? Should we be concerned when a women has a less than positive birth experience as long as her child is healthy? Do the routine interventions at hospitals today _really_ save infants' lives? More and more research shows that they do not. It seems then that what is really at issue is a woman's power and her ability to realize that power during birth. When a woman gives birth without the aid of drugs or anesthesia she suddenly realizes how really strong she is. Her husband will also realize this and it may be a scary thing for him, especially if he has always thought of his wife as a weak woman who must be protected. But when we take away birth from women, saving them from pain, rescuing them from the hard work of labor, we also prevent them from growing as people.

Women who give birth vaginally without anesthesia or other drugs have overcome one of life's more difficult challenges.
Getting through labor is a test of character, determination, strength and will. But it is infinitely easier to do when an experienced woman is leading the way. A woman who has given birth herself, a woman who trusts in the birth process as the best and right way to bring children into the world, a woman who knows that birth is a sacred, transcendent experience. This special woman is the professional labor assistant. She can help mothers have a birth experience that will last them a lifetime. She can make the difference between a joyous time when new life enters the world, or a frightening, overwhelming, out-of-control experience.

People in our country, in our culture, view birth as a medical emergency, an event that women must be "saved from." Many women begin their pregnancies with painful images of labor in the back of their minds. If they have friends who have given birth, they will likely relate tales of medical interventions, anesthesia, all of which will further validate their beliefs that birth is a difficult and painful affair. Childbirth education classes offered by most hospitals often bury the fact that pain is a normal part of birth. This may further the image of mechanized birth as usual, acceptable, and therefore, best. Husbands and wives faithfully practice their breathing techniques, believing that this will help with the pain during labor.

When labor actually begins, many women (and their husbands) are unprepared for the reality of birth, and almost immediately will want relief from what they interpret as unusual or unnecessary pain. Since most doctors and nurses on obstetrical wards rarely see an unmedicated, natural birth they will provide that pain relief to the mother, even though there are plenty of non-medical techniques that can help a mother to cope. And even as she is numbed from anesthesia, the mother (and father) may wonder why she "failed" to have natural childbirth. These mothers will not have the experience of testing the limits of their body's endurance, their mind's ability to cope, or their own vision of personal strength. They will not grow as much as if they had participated fully in their birth experience. It is no wonder that after birth, many women feel that something is missing. It is often puzzling to them that even when their labor was normal, there were no complications, and their baby was healthy, that they lack a feeling of completeness.

Western Culture Ignores Wisdom of the Ages

Our highly "advanced" country is one of the few cultures that does not provide someone to continuously care for the laboring mother. . In order to help a woman feel more confident, the job of nurses, midwives, obstetricians, family practitioners, professional labor assistants such as doulas and monitrices, childbirth educators, perinatologists, pediatricians, and neonatalogist entails empowerment and building self-esteem while educating the mother about ways to keep both her and her baby safe. The environment in which the birth takes place has an equally dynamic effect on the life of the mother and baby. It is important to create an atmosphere in the birth room where a mother feels safe. Our care should build on the woman's strengths not emphasize her weaknesses. It is the sense of feeling safe and trusting those around her that gives the mother the confidence she needs to birth her own baby. In one study of 128 cultures in non-industrialized countries, 126 provide for the presence of a woman with the mother during the entire labor and birth. During the first one third of the labor, this social support person is close to the mother, touches her, hugs her, and holds her hands. During the last one third of the labor she literally holds the mother in her arms. Seventy nine percent of the time, she is within one foot of the mother.[1]

The role of this special woman who mothers the mother during birth has been largely missing from the birth scene of North America. Even though many fathers are now present in the delivery room, a father can't know what pain his wife is experiencing because he has never done what she is doing. And even if the labor nurse in attendance is herself a mother, she is often on a shift schedule and may leave just when the mother has gotten used to her and needs her most. But now there are two kinds of professional women who are filling this role of continuous care for the laboring mother--doulas, from the Greek, meaning "in service of," and monitrices, from the French, meaning "to watch over." Doulas provide physical and emotional support during birth, but do no assessment of fetal or maternal well-being. Monitrices who combine nurturing with clinical skills. Both doulas and monitrices are increasingly involved in providing labor support in birth in our culture and are commonly referred to as professional labor assistants. The doula or monitrice is there to support not only the mother but her partner as well. She is an integral part of making the birth environment a trusting one for all concerned.

Researchers Prove What Women Know

What women have known over the ages is now being documented by modern, scientific researchers studying birthing women. Before the 1920's it was common in North America to have a woman companion present during labor and birth. After that time, the focus on maternity then turned more to relieving the pain of childbirth with medications thus resulting in childbirth being an "emotionally isolating event for many women."(12) The benefits of a continuous labor assistant were studied by Marshall Klaus, M.D. and John Kennell, M.D. Since their original studies in the 1980's, there have been eleven scientific trials conducted in many countries comparing usual care with usual care plus attendance of a doula. The studies found that in hospitals where intervention rates (epidural anesthesia, oxytocin, forceps delivery, and cesarean sections) were high, doula care lowered the intervention rates. (1-6) All six trials that investigated postpartum outcomes (breastfeeding, maternal infant interaction, postpartum depression, anxiety, self-esteem, maternal assessments of their baby when compared to the "standard baby," and satisfaction with the birth experience) found that women who had doulas had these more positive outcomes four to eight weeks later than those without doulas. (1,7-11)The continuous social support during labor significantly reduces the incidence of medical interventions, reduces the incidence of neonatal complications and maternal fevers, and shortens the length of labor.

From the Klaus and Kennell research, it is quite clear that not only are mothers and babies benefiting, but health care costs are decreased dramatically. One study calculated that the cost savings for individual families was approximately $3,500 showing that a doula program is a benefit not only to families, nurses, and hospitals but to third party carriers as well. With conservative estimates the comparison of 100 births with a doula shows a cost savings of $15,000.

The skills of the professional labor assistant are combined with the expertise of physicians, midwives, and nurses thus improving perinatal outcomes for both mothers and their infants. Both types of labor professionals:

- stay with the laboring woman continuously
- believe that women are strong and capable
- are aware that births are significant life events
- are aware that labor and delivery are normal physiological processes as well as an emotional, social, sexual and spiritual life events
- understand the emotional needs of the laboring woman
- are knowledgeable about the anatomy and physiology of labor and birth
- have expertise in comfort measures and coping skills necessary during the birth process
- provide an objective viewpoint
- can act as a liaison and facilitate communication with other health care professionals
- believe that pregnant couples should have trust in their caregivers
- help strengthen the relationship between the mother and her partner
- believe that decisions about pregnancy, labor and birth should be made by the pregnant couple with input from health care professionals
- understand that birth is a life altering event for the woman
- support the decisions of the mother and her partner
- respect the mother's individuality and uniqueness
- trust mothers and their partners to have the ability to make the best decisions for themselves and their babies
- help create positive birth memories

The professional labor assistant is emerging as a positive contribution to maternity care. Besides reducing medical costs and risks of anesthesia or surgery, professional labor assistants bring humane care back to one of life's most important events, birth.

References:
[1] Sosa R, et al, "The effect of a supportive companion on perinatal problems, length of labor, and mother-infant interaction," *N Engl J Med*, 303:597-600, 1980.

[2] Klaus MH, et al, "Effects of social support during parturition on maternal and infant morbidity, "" *Br Med J*, 293:585-587, 1986.

[3] Kennell JH, et al, "Continuous emotional support during labor in a US

hospital: a randomized controlled trail, "" *JAMA*, 265:2197-2201, 1991.

[4.] Hodnett ED, et al, "Effects of continuous intrapartum professional of childbirth outcomes, " *Res in Nursing and Health*, 12:287-289, 1989.

[5.] Kennell JH, et al, "Labor support by a doula for middle-income couple: the effect on cesarean rates, " *Pediatric Res*, 32:12A, 1993.

[6.] McGrath SK, et al, "Induction of labor and doula support, " *Pediatric Res*, 43:13A, 1998.

[7.] Garcia C, "The eighth doula study: social support during birth in Mexico, Conference proceedings of Doulas of North America, Austin, TX, June 20,1997, 89-93.

[8.] Hofmeyr J, et al, "Companionship to modify the clinical birth environment: effects of perceptions of labour and breastfeeding, " *Br J Obstet Gynaecol*, 98:756-764, 1991.

[9.] Landry SH, et al, "The effects of doula support during labor on mother-infant interaction at two months, "" *Pediatric Res*, 43:13A, 1998.

[10.] Walton D, et al, "The impact of hospital based doula program in a health maintenance organization setting, "" *Am J Obstet Gyncol*, 11, 1998.

[11.] Wolman WL, et al, "Postpartum depression and companionship in the clinical birth environment: a randomized, controlled study, "" *Am J Obstet Gyncol*, 168:1388-1393, 1993.

[12.] Scott KD, et al, "The Obstetrical and Postpartum Benefits of Continuous Support during Childbirth," *J of Women's Health & Gender-Based Medicine*, 8(10): 1257-1264, 1999.

2.
Why Parents Need Professional Labor Support

"The laboring woman needs total support in order to let go completely to allow her system to respond to the power of the birthing process."

Phyllis Klaus

Although vaginal births constitute the majority of births in this country, those births are usually "managed births" with a host of medical, technological, interventions of questionable necessity. Only ten percent of the 3.5 million American women who give birth each year do so without intervention. With that reality, it's not surprising that women desiring natural birth in a hospital setting increasingly choose to hire a professional labor assistants.

"My first daughter was born by cesarean section. Her birth was disastrous. My husband and I felt very victimized by the medical community and I grieved for the lost experience of birthing my baby. Our labor assistant for our second birth helped us deal with the trauma of the first birth."

"Now I know that sometimes unnecessary or risky interventions can be avoided if a knowledgeable person asks the right questions. If only someone had been there to help me ask the right questions."

"I believe no woman should labor without a caring woman with her."

"When I went to the hospital I was hooked up to a fetal monitor, flat on my back, and my waters were broken. Even though my husband gave me terrific support, after 6cm, I couldn't cope. I received an epidural and shortly after that the fetal heartbeat started slowing down with contractions. At 8cm the staff started talking about the possibility of a cesarean which wouldn't be decided upon until I was in the O.R. The staff decided I would have a cesarean. I felt as if I wasn't part of the situation and my husband was left outside until after the birth."

"When the cesarean section decision was made. I was so sad. Reed had left to go get our camera and the nurses were rushing around in a frenzy. I felt incredibly alone and sad. Polly leaned down by my head and spoke so calmly. She told me what a wonderful job I had done and how proud I should be of myself. I was crying, but she kept right on talking. By the time

I got to the delivery room, I was happy and excited. It's amazing how she lifted me out of such despair."

"During my second birth, I was screaming for medication and felt at that point that a cesarean was the easy way out. Although I begged for an epidural, Janice and my husband helped me continue. It was just a cry for help. I was really tired. I needed encouragement, not drugs."

"I was very excited that I had done it, that it was another boy, that I had pushed the baby out, and that I HAD GIVEN BIRTH!"

"Having labor support at a birth is a must! Brian and I both agree that if we had had someone with us at Shannon's birth it might have been just what we needed to give us the extra time so that we could have had Shannon vaginally. I don't think the 5 oz. between Shannon who was 10 pounds and Patrick who was 9lb.11 oz. made that much difference."

"John and I will never forget the monitrice and her calm ways and soft and encouraging voice. I gained much strength from her presence and her faith in me. I see now that she spoke the truth. Since she spoke with wisdom and care I know it was right to trust her. It still astounds me what support and confidence from others can do for a person. I could never have done it as well on my own. Now the birth of my first son will outshine all memories-past and future."

"I was sent to a high risk referral hospital where I was delivered by c-section under emergency circumstances at 32   1/2 weeks. The baby was taken immediately to the neonatal intensive care unit after only a brief glance at him by his parents. My husband was allowed to see him again after being robed and masked but I was unable to see or hold him until 24 hours later."

"I was disappointed when my son was taken to the nursery immediately after birth. My labor assistant quickly suggested that I be rolled in a wheelchair to the nursery to sit by his side. The nurse agreed and I "recovered" in the nursery. I'm afraid that if my labor assistant hadn't been there, no one would have suggested that alternative and I would have unnecessarily missed being with my son during his first few hours of life."

"The pushing process went very quickly. The help of the monitrice was especially good at this point as the labor nurse was so busy filling out

papers that she couldn't help me until after the birth. Neither my husband nor I could have done it without the help of the monitrice."

"We were so thrilled to have Laura and without a monitrice there I am afraid that she would never have turned and I would have had another cesarean. Without the encouragement we got from the monitrice and the faith we had in her, the story of Laura's birth would have been entirely different."

Professional labor support can mean the difference between a good birth experience, and a disastrous, demeaning, or disappointing birth experience. This is the central reason motivated, educated, couples have given for choosing professional labor support. First time parents often need the extra confidence a labor assistant can provide. Her presence can help reduce their fear, clumsiness, and vulnerability. These couples feel their chances of giving birth without the use of drugs and unnecessary interventions are better with the extra support the labor assistant can provide.

"During our childbirth classes we came to feel that we wanted to minimize intervention, especially pain medication during labor. Though our classes helped instill in us the confidence to pursue natural childbirth, we felt that the support of an experienced skilled caregiver would greatly assist us with our decision."

A Help to Fathers

Men are choosing to take an increasingly active role in the process of labor and birth. They attend childbirth and parenting classes and remain with their partners during the birth process. This is generally viewed as satisfying and beneficial for all. However, many men find that along with this participation comes increased expectations of them. They are sometimes expected to be the "labor authority" when they do not feel qualified for that role. First time fathers realize their wives may need more reassurance, support and guidance than they can provide. Experienced or not, fathers may need the relief and help that a labor assistant can bring to the long hours of labor. They are anxious to support and nurture their partners, but realize their expertise with birth is limited to the knowledge gained in childbirth classes or to their own previous attendance at birth. Men have feelings of insecurity in labor and need support and guidance.

"We hired a monitrice to take the pressure off my husband as labor authority so that he could focus on being involved in the birth experience."

"I knew my husband could help me but I worried about what would happen if we both panicked."

The labor assistant acknowledges that fathers may have many anxieties about their role in labor. Her presence allows the father to direct his attention to loving and supporting the laboring mother while feeling loved and supported too.

"We felt that my husband needed the support, guidance, and relief a monitrice could provide."

The labor assistant's deep and encompassing trust in the birth process and her objectivity helps keep both parents balanced during this emotional time. Her presence may help some fathers cope while seeing their wives in pain. Her knowledge and acceptance of pain as part of the birth process may help the father who feels the need to rescue his wife from pain.

"As the labor assistant, I am not nearly as emotionally involved as the father is. I know that contractions open the cervix; I have been with women in pain and I know that it doesn't kill them. I have a degree of objectivity that the dad doesn't."

Home Care Before Going to the Hospital

Many couples do not want to go to the hospital in early labor but want access to skilled care at home. They may be concerned about their ability to determine when it is appropriate to go to the hospital. The labor assistant can assess the signs of active labor depending on her training, and may do vaginal exams, while the couple stays at home during early labor. Her presence sets their minds at ease and helps them avoid the "too early" trip to the hospital. The monitrice can also keep the parents informed about the well-being of the baby, by listening to and interpreting fetal heart tones. A doula does not perform any clinical assessments of mother or baby. She relies on the same signs that the mother relies on in deciding when to go to the hospital--contractions, status of membranes, subjective feelings.

"We wanted to labor at home as long as possible with the confidence that dilatation was progressing and the baby was well."

"I wanted to labor at home yet did not want to jeopardize my baby's or my health."

Parents may want the person who cared for them at home to continue that care at the hospital. Labor assistants are also helpful to the couple who choose to give birth at home, and to the midwife or doctor who provides home birth care.

A Help to Nurses, Midwives and Doctors

Once they get to the hospital, couples may have another worry. It is a well-publicized fact that there is a nursing shortage in the United States, and in some hospitals, the nursing vacancy rates are in the double digits. Sometimes inexperienced nurses fill in. Sometimes nurses have to care for more than one woman at a time. Sometimes they can offer only minimal care. For these reasons, couples may worry about the quality of nursing care they will receive. The labor assistant can be of help to the nursing staff and to doctors and midwives.

There are other limitations to a hospital delivery that the labor assistant can mitigate. Hospital nurses are unknown, unchosen individuals to the couple, while the labor assistant is usually hand picked in advance. Nurses in hospitals work eight to twelve hour shifts, and during an average length labor, the family might have several nurses in attendance. A mother can come to depend on one nurse, only to have her or him leave at a crucial time in the labor because of a shift change.

"We hired a labor assistant to avoid the interruptions caused by different shifts of nurses."

"I wanted someone I chose, not someone chosen for me."

Unlike the hospital nurse on a shift, the labor assistant remains with the couple throughout the labor and birth. She will aid them, guide them and keep them informed of the progression of the labor.

"Once I had hired the monitrice I knew I would have someone experienced there all the time."

When the mother isn't worried about the shift system in the hospital she is more able to take advantage of the care that the hospital nurses can provide. Knowing that her labor assistant will always be with her allows her to continue laboring undisturbed by nurses changing shifts, taking breaks, etc. If her labor assistant has worked previously with the nursing staff it will be easier for the mother to accept care from this person she has never met before.

Couples may also be concerned that the nurse will have a stronger commitment to the hospital's rules and regulations and "ways of doing things" than to their needs. This can and does present a conflict of interests. Couples are also concerned that the nurse may be more anxious to please the doctor than them. A professional labor assistant has a commitment only to the laboring couple and their baby. Nurses find that the presence of the professional labor assistant helps them avoid many sticky situations where there could be a conflict between the regulations and the wants of the couple.

"When the hospital nurse hugged my labor assistant and said 'I'm so glad to see you again, it's such fun when your clients come in,' I knew everything would be okay."

Philosophy of Care

Families may also be concerned that the hospital staff will not share their philosophy of birth. This is very likely if the parents want a natural birth and live in an area where the majority of vaginal births are medically managed. Birth in many areas of the United States is synonymous with epidural anesthesia, continuous electronic fetal monitoring, episiotomy, and forceps delivery. By hiring someone independent of the hospital, a couple is able to assure they will be cared for by someone who shares a commitment to natural birth with as little intervention as possible. Often the presence of the labor assistant helps identify to the staff the couples that want a unmedicated birth. This helps the staff when assignments are made when the couple arrives at the hospital.

"I wanted someone with medical training who would be at the birth to give advice consistent with my philosophy of birthing."

"I felt the need for a loving, experienced professional that shared my beliefs on birthing and would encourage me to birth as I had planned."
"I figured I would do all I could to try and have a natural delivery."

Fetal monitoring may seem to take priority in the birth. Experienced mothers may hire labor support to prevent the occurrence of problems or unpleasant events that occurred during a previous birth.

"During my first birth, although the nurses were kind and competent they seemed more concerned with the technology than with my needs."

Avoiding a Cesarean

With the national percentages of cesarean birth hovering at 25% and individual hospitals having rates above fifty percent, parents are justifiably concerned. They feel the presence of a professional labor assistant will lower the chances of an unnecessary cesarean.

"I had a fear of an unnecessary cesarean. I felt having another professional there to represent my interests to the physician at a time when I myself might not be clearly heard would make me more at ease."

The Help of Another Woman

For many years and in many cultures, the relationship of other experienced women to a laboring woman was respected. Many women still feel it is important to have another woman with them during labor, a woman with experience or who has given birth herself.

"We were uneasy with the thought of laboring without someone who had been through it before."

Another mother can provide support in a way that no one else can. She has traveled a similar road, and that simple fact gives the laboring mother vital emotional support. She has the ability to provide comfort by knowing support is needed before the mother asks for it. When the contractions are intense and the journey seems endless it is often important for the mother to know that she is being taken care of by another woman who has been through the birth experience. This wisdom of the ages helps laboring mothers tremendously.

"I wanted to be able to see in your eyes and feel in your touch that you knew what I was going through."

"I am there to help them just like their mother or father was when they learned to ride a bicycle. During birth I am the parent who held on to the back of the bicycle until the rider had some experience and felt safe and turned around to see that they had been riding on their own for quite some time."

Birth as a Peak Experience

Many parents today realize that birth is one of the peak experiences in their lives and they choose caregivers who will enhance this experience with individualized care.

"We knew this would probably be our only birth experience and wanted it to be a once in a lifetime thing."

Families know that with the help of professional labor support they will be more confident, more relaxed and more able to fully appreciate their birth experience.

"We hired professional labor support because we wanted to maximize our birth experience."

"We hired the monitrice as insurance that the birth would go as planned and because we liked the monitrice as a person."

First time parents especially, hire a labor assistant because they want to minimize their anxiety of the unknown.

"We needed the support of somebody who cared to be with us, especially with our first child. We have used the same monitrice for all three of our children."

Special Needs

Numerous individual reasons encourage families to choose professional labor support. Those may include parents having a vaginal birth after cesarean (VBAC), single mothers, teenage mothers, mothers with multiple pregnancies and mothers with hypertension or diabetes.

"When my gestational diabetes was diagnosed, I thought my plans for a natural birth would have to go out the window. My labor assistant told me she'd cared for many people with diabetes who were able to birth without interventions. She helped me stick to my diet. She was right: I had a natural birth."

"My monitrice gave me lots of information about how to control my blood pressure. She discussed things about diet that my doctor never mentioned."

Those who desire a vaginal birth after a previous cesarean birth (VBAC) are very concerned about preventing another cesarean. They want someone who trusts the normal birth process, someone who will not be afraid of the fact that the woman has had a cesarean.

"We hired her to give additional emotional support. We knew that mothers who have had cesareans sometimes need more support because of that experience."

Single mothers may have no close friends or family with whom they choose to share the birth. The professional labor assistant may be their only or best support.

"Since I was single and pregnant I was so excited when our Lamaze teacher talked about professional labor assistants. I jumped at the chance to hire a monitrice."

Mothers with obstetrical risks are greatly helped by having a labor assistant present during their birth. It is often necessary for the nurses' attention to be focused on the technology necessary to insure safe delivery.

"Since I was having twins, I wanted someone around who would think about me. It seemed everyone except my husband and my labor assistant focused only on the twins."

Some primary caregivers may recommend or require the services of a professional labor support person. Nursing personnel in the hospital may recommend such services to those who they feel have inadequate support when they enter the hospital. Parents may want someone to act as their advocate; someone who can intercede on their behalf if that becomes necessary. Some hospitals have found that hospital doula programs are helpful to not only the pregnant couple but to the hospital staff as well.

"We hired a monitrice because we wanted an advocate to represent us during our time in the hospital in case there was any last minute dispute over our birth plan."

A father's out of town business travel scheduled close to the due date may prompt some to seek professional help. A father who is in the armed services may find himself on a ship or temporary duty away from home during the latter part of the pregnancy. A father may have been transferred to another city, while his wife remains home. A monitrice can provide reassurance to the father that his wife will be in good hands if he is unable to get back in time for the birth.

"When we found out that I might be out of town when our second child was due we hired someone we knew we could count on to be with my wife."

Families who want to involve their children in the birth process find it helpful to have a professional person present who is experienced and comfortable with children. The labor assistant often teaches the children prenatally and then in the labor helps integrate the children into the birth experience.

"I hired a monitrice so that my children could attend the birth of their sibling."

Couples who have used professional support once often come back for assistance again. The couple who has used a professional labor assistant hires her as soon as the pregnancy is confirmed.

"We had used the monitrice for our first birth and we couldn't imagine not having her there for the second birth."

"For my second pregnancy I knew that I needed all the support I could get. We used the monitrice the first time and had a good experience. We felt that if the monitrice had not been present at our first birth I would have had a cesarean section."

Couples may be unfamiliar with the health care system and feel that a professional labor support person will help them in what they see as an alien, threatening world.

"We wanted a patient advocate as we were unfamiliar with routine procedures in this country and were afraid of unnecessary medical intervention. This all seemed more important as we had just recently moved to Houston from Canada."

Couples with a language barrier benefit from having someone present who is familiar with their language or who can make sure others understand them.

"We had just moved here from Germany and were having trouble communicating in English. We hired a monitrice because we knew that she would always take the time to be sure that we understood what was

happening. We had already had problems with people speaking too rapidly for us to understand."

Teenage mothers often need extra support and reassurance.

"My doula never talked down to me and always treated me like an adult. This helped me learn mothering skills."

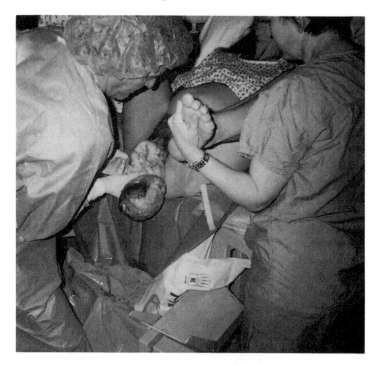

The labor assistant provides support in many ways.

How Parents Should Choose a Labor Assistant

Once a couple decides to hire a professional labor assistant, they should interview prospective support persons carefully, considering her background and training, her relationship with the medical community, the number of births she has attended, the types of clients she has cared for, her experience with complications, the limits of her practice, her fees, and her backup arrangements or call schedule. Besides professional considerations, the couple will want to find out if the labor support person has values compatible with their own and personal qualities they desire. These might include honesty, patience, flexibility, credibility, good communication skills, self confidence, advocacy skills, sensitivity, availability, sense of humor, empathy, lack of prejudice, warmth, tenderness, a supportive caring nature, respect for the birth process, and a love for women.

Interview Questions

When choosing a labor assistant, answers to the following questions will help parents find the right support person.

- What type of practice do you have? Doula, Labor Support, Monitrice, Midwife?
- What is your educational background?
- How did you receive your training as a Labor Support Person?
- Do you give care for births in the hospital? At a birth center? At home?
- How many births have you attended? Over what time span? What is your average number of births per month?
- What type of clients have you cared for? Who is your backup? When might they care for me?
- What are your fees? When do I need to pay the fee? Do you have a sliding scale? Will you barter for the fee?
- Will I be able to get third part reimbursement for your services?
- Do you restrict your practice in any way?
- When would I call you? Can I reach you 24 hours a day?
- Will you come to my home when I'm in labor?
- How will you know if a complication arises while I'm laboring at home?
- Do you listen to and interpret the fetal heart tones?
- Do you do vaginal examinations?
- How do you determine maternal well-being during labor?
- What is your relationship with hospital/birth center personnel?
- Have you ever worked with my physician/midwife? What was that experience like?
- Are any restrictions placed on you by the hospital/birth center? If so, what are they?
- Do you get along well with the hospital staff or my doctor? Have you had any conflict with them? If yes, do you think it will interfere with your ability to help me?
- If someone suggests an intervention that you feel is unnecessary what will you do or say?
- How can you help us minimize the need for an episiotomy?
- If I need a cesarean will you be able to accompany me?
- Have you ever cared for anyone with a poor outcome? What was the situation?

- What do you provide that is different from what the hospital/birth center staff can provide?
- What do you provide that is different than what my partner can provide?
- What do you provide that is different than what my physician/midwife can provide?
- Why did you become a professional labor support person?
- What do you like best about your job?
- What do you like least about your job?
- Why do you feel labor support is helpful?
- May I have references of others you have cared for?

If you are planning to be a professional birth assistant, think about how you will answer such questions and be prepared to clarify these matters in an interview even if your prospective clients do not initiate these questions.

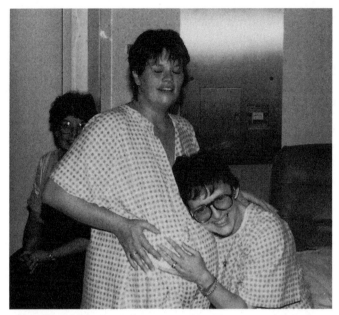

Humor helps the mother keep her perspective. It can help the monitrice too.

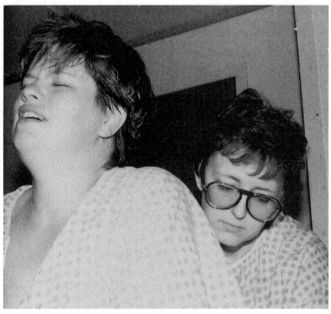

Labor is hard work for the mother...and the labor assistant too.

3.
Why Women Want to be Labor Assistants and the Reality of the Job They Choose

Labor assistants come to this profession for a variety of reasons. Many decide to get involved after the birth of their own child. That highly emotional experience, whether positive or negative, is a strong motivational factor. These women have come to deeply understand the need for support during labor and birth, and they hope to help other women achieve a good birth and avoid a traumatic birth.

"My own birth experiences-a cesarean 9 years ago with only my husband in attendance and then two VBAC's (one in the hospital and one at home) with husband, midwife and many friends in attendance-- convinced me that the laboring couple can work together more effectively if they are supported by knowledgeable, loving people who are totally committed to them and no one else at the time of their labor."

"When I became pregnant with my first child I researched, read and interviewed more than I ever imagined I would. I worked hard for the birth I wanted and it was worth every moment. After the birth of my daughter I felt a joy I had never known before. At that time I decided to seek out helping other women."

"During my own labor, my husband was too tired and anxious to help me and I spent many immobile hours alone. This resulted in a tremendously negative experience and I felt I never could give birth again. Later I realized it was the support and caring that was missing."

"My births were so impersonal and nearly tragic in one instance that I felt it had to be better than what I had been involved in. I felt that with training I could help others have the births I did not have."

"I decided to become a labor support person because I had a labor assistant myself with my second birth and had not had one with the first. The differences in the two births were unbelievable. I enjoyed my second birth where my first birth had nightmare qualities. I decided I wanted to help others to make labor more enjoyable and drug free."

For some labor support professionals, helping women through birth is a calling. It is not just something they choose to do; it is something they must do. It is not uncommon to hear labor support providers say, "How can I not do this?"

"I had the knowledge and felt the need to share the supporting role I can play."

"I felt a calling to do this. I feel a real and deep need to help."

Some feel this calling in a more spiritual sense.

"I believe that God led me into doing this for women. It has   been a special ministry that is under his divine guidance."

Some doulas and monitrices have chosen this profession because of their strong bond with other women. They feel there is a strong need for women to be helped by other women during this time of birth. They feel their presence helps the mother to recognize and appreciate her link with all other mothers--those who have birthed before and those who have yet to birth. The labor assistant is their link with time; this link helps the mother to know that she too can birth her baby. She too has the wisdom of the ages.

Nurses as Professional Labor Assistants

Some nurses go into labor support as a natural progression from their work in the maternity care field. Labor and delivery nurses often become professional labor support persons in order to make better use of their talents. They may have felt too restricted as an employee of the hospital. They may have had to leave a woman at a critical point in her labor once too often. Nurses often see mothers who come to the hospital too early in labor; they know that if they had had someone knowledgeable with them at home, they would have waited and come to the hospital at a more appropriate time. They find they can use their talents more effectively if they are able to focus on the physical, emotional, and spiritual comfort of the mother rather than the medical-legal-political issues that their role as a hospital staff nurse dictates. Being dedicated to one couple only--not to the couple and the physician and the hospital--gives them a clearer role definition.

"When I was an OB nurse I saw that too many women did not believe in themselves, in their bodies and in their ability to do the thing that women

have been doing for centuries-give birth. I realized I could focus on empowering women much better as a monitrice."

"I saw some wonderful birthing experiences in labor and delivery, but unless the patient was also a very close personal friend, I would wish her luck and leave her to the next shift. All too often this was during her transition time. Now, as a monitrice, I am able to stay and not leave her just when she needs me the most."

"Working as a nurse, saw many couples who were vulnerable and afraid. They could have done just fine if they had had a supportive person with them who knew them and knew the kind of birth they wanted."

From the Ranks of Childbirth Educators

Most professional labor assistants are also childbirth educators. Their work in childbirth education has shown them the realities of the health care system. They see many couples who suffer from not being supported. They are concerned about the students they teach, especially in areas where the hospitals and caregivers do not offer family-centered care. They move into this role as a way of continuing the education and support that began in their childbirth classes.

"I see labor support as a portion of my role as a childbirth educator."

"I moved gradually from being a Bradley Method teacher into labor support."

"As a childbirth educator I got tired of 'sending the lambs to the slaughter' and decided to give my students the one-to-one support they needed."

Another reason for the preponderance of childbirth educators among labor assistants is that the training of a childbirth educator often involves the observation of labors and births. The chance to see births other than their own and to see the big difference that labor support can make often prompts them to seek out training as labor support professionals. Others find that labor support is a step in their midwifery education. Some use labor assisting as a way of deciding whether they want to pursue midwifery while others use it as the first or second step in their midwifery education.

"During my observations of laboring women, required for certification of childbirth educators in this city, I noticed how many men, although willing, were frightened and withdrawn during labor. When I was allowed to help with support, the man would immediately regain his confidence and be of help."

"My decision to be a labor assistant grew originally out of my strong feeling of exhilaration, before during and after the births I observed during my ASPO training. The entire process fascinated me and the incredible feelings of being in touch with the woman/couple was so special."

Education

The educational background of labor assistants can vary and will determine the level of care the assistant can provide. Nurses or midwives bring an educational background that includes didactic information about pregnancy and birth as well as the clinical skills to assess the physical well-being of both mother and child. Childbirth educators, if certified, have a background that includes required reading, educational seminars, class observations, birth observations, and a written test or syllabus. Content areas for testing include conception and pregnancy, nutrition, labor, birth and post-partum, professional responsibility, instructional methods and teaching skills, emotional aspects of pregnancy, obstetrical procedures, cesarean birth, and labor coping skills. Certified childbirth educators are expected to remain current in their field. Certifying bodies required recertification periodically every few years. The recertification process often includes birth observations, attendance at continuing education workshops, and class evaluations. Lamaze, International, Inc., The American Society for Psychoprophylaxis in Obstetrics (ASPO), The American Academy of Husband-Coached Childbirth, The International Childbirth Education Association, Birthworks, and Association of Labor Assistants and Childbirth Educators (addresses in "Resources" at the end of the book) are some of the nation-wide or international organizations that train and certify childbirth educators.

Training Programs

With formal education as a foundation, training for the role of labor assistant or monitrice incorporates an apprenticeship, on the job training, and occasionally a formal labor support or birth assistant training program such as those offered by Childbirth Enhancement Foundation, Doulas of North America, International Childbirth

Education Association, and Lamaze, Inc.(See addresses in "Resources" at the end of the book.)

The more comprehensive the service provided by the labor assistant the more comprehensive the training should be. If the labor assistant is offering only emotional support and assistance with labor coping skills it is not necessary that her training include clinical nursing or midwifery skills for fetal and maternal assessment. However, the more comprehensive monitrice services require training in the following skills: assessment and interpretation of maternal temperature, pulse, respiration and blood pressure; reading of urine test sticks, Leopold's maneuvers to identify presentation, position, attitude, variety and lie; measurement of fundal height; fetal heart rate determination and interpretation; enema administration; vaginal examination to identify cervical dilatation, effacement and position of cervix, station of presenting part, and fetal position and attitude; conduct and interpretation of a home non-stress test; eliciting and assessment of deep tendon reflexes (DTR) and clonus; administration and assessment nitrazine test; and response to fetal distress.

The Reality of 24 Hour Call

Before becoming a professional labor assistant one must consider the reality of 24 hour call. Pregnant women and their families need help around the clock, not just from nine to five. Being on call can mean working on Christmas Eve or your child's birthday. It can mean leaving in the middle of a school program or missing a family celebration entirely.

"In the past eight years I have helped mothers birth babies on every major holiday, my birthday, my husband's birthday, and all of my children's birthdays. I have tried to include my family in these births by telling about the birth and the baby. Now my children see the births I attend, even at holidays, birthdays, and celebrations, as very special babies born on very special days."

Being a professional labor assistant is not just a job; it is a way of life. It means the possibility of working long hours; much longer than the usual eight hour work day. Therefore, not only must the labor assistant be committed to her profession but so must the rest of her family. It requires dedication, organization, communication, flexibility, and infinite patience from everyone. Most professional labor assistants do not share a practice; they are on call all the time except for very special occasions or out of town trips. The best way for them to have time for themselves is to limit the number of clients they take and to space their due dates far enough apart to give themselves a break. Some, however, work in partnerships and organizations that allow labor assistants to share call or work a designated shift. The mother hires the organization and whoever is on call will assist her. This may mean that the mother does not meet the labor assistant prior to labor. In small partnerships, however, the couple usually gets to know all the labor assistants prior to the birth.

Being on call means not only being on call for births but for phone calls. It is a reality that families sometimes need your advice or assistance during supper, in the middle of the night, and even during love-making! An understanding and supportive mate makes this on call situation much more livable. Family survival requires open honest communication.

"We don't let the fact that my wife is on call run our lives. We still purchase theater tickets and plan family outings. The worst that happens is that my wife cannot go; I still go to the theater-sometimes with someone else-and the family still goes on the outings."

Unfortunately, many labor assistants abandon their practice after working for a while. They burn out, often because they took on too many clients and were not prepared for the impact of the job on their lives. Being a labor assistant not just a job it is a life choice. The demands of labor support as a full-time profession are often too great for those with small children. These are the unpleasant realities that must be faced before entering into the profession.

"I worked as a monitrice for two and a half years and gave it up. It was too difficult on my husband and small children for me to be on call. I still occasionally do labor support for a friend although my family discourages me."

"I worked as a monitrice for two and a half years and gave it up. It was too difficult on my husband and small children for me to be on call. I still occasionally do labor support for a friend although my family discourages me."

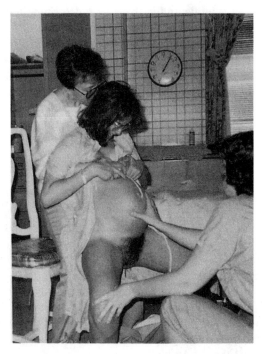

Being a labor assistant can be an exhausting job.

Support for the Labor Assistant

A good support system is another requirement for this demanding role. The labor assistant needs someone who can be called in the middle of a difficult labor or when she is frustrated with herself or other caregivers; someone who understands. Participating in study groups not only provides a way to increase one's knowledge; it also provides a way to give and receive support. Involvement with a local childbirth educator's organization or midwifery organization is another way to broaden one's support system. At the very least the labor assistant needs ONE person she can call at 3am when she's upset, confused, excited, or needs advice--someone who understands, who will listen well and give wise counsel.

Before becoming a professional labor assistant, one must consider the emotional outlay involved in this profession. It requires a tremendous amount of giving. In many ways, what we do is intense mothering, and as any mother knows, we often have to give to those in our care even when we are not sure we have anything left to give. We must give to our clients in many ways, emotionally, physically, and spiritually.   Walt Whitman might have been describing the professional labor assistant when he wrote, *"When I give, I give myself."*

Because of this, the labor assistant needs to learn how to receive as well as to give. Those of us who choose this profession are often very good at giving, but may need to learn much about receiving without guilt. We must learn how to receive from others in order to keep ourselves strong, or we may reach a point where we are no longer able to give. One must keep her own cup full if she is going to constantly be refilling others' cups.

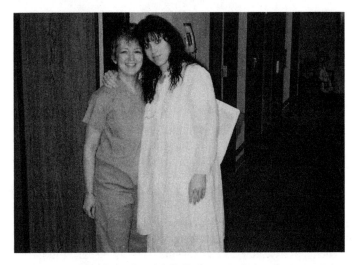

The labor assistant's belief in the woman's strength
helps her believe in herself.

Not for Everyone

Being a professional labor assistant is not a profession for someone who wants to be "in charge." A labor assistant or monitrice is there to serve women and their families, not control their births. She is not there to tell women how to have their babies, but to help them find their own individual ways to give birth. Labor assistants know that birth is a process which can span from A to Z and that not all mothers get from one point to the other in the same way. The monitrice's job is to lift some of the stumbling blocks along the way so that the process is facilitated, not hindered. It is not for her to direct the mother but to be a support along side her. She is there to help provide safe passage for both mother and babe. She is not there to try to make the physician or hospital conform to her way of thinking; she is there to support the families' wishes. She should not project her own desires on the couple but should present them with clear, honest information with which they will make their own choices.

"I sometimes have to swallow hard and support the mother in something I personally would not have chosen. Just the other night I had a client who insisted on an epidural, even with all my encouragement and reminders that she was progressing well. The bottom line is that it is her body, her birth experience, and her baby. I (reluctantly) helped her to get the epidural."

Just as parents trust the birth assistant to care for them she should trust their ability to make the right decisions for themselves and their baby. When events take an unexpected turn during the labor and birth, the labor assistant can help the couple see that all is not lost. She can help highlight those issues over which they still have some control or decision making.

The Possibility of an Unexpected Home Birth

If you are doing labor support at home, prior to a planned hospital birth, you must recognize the possibility, albeit small, that labor will progress so rapidly that the mother cannot be transported to the hospital. You may also encounter a laboring mother who refuses to be taken to the hospital, even though she originally planned to a hospital birth. It is not within the scope of this book to prepare you to attend a birth as the primary caregiver. However, if you assist a laboring woman at home, you should ask yourself these questions:

- Is your training sufficient to permit you to assist laboring women at home?
- Do I have the necessary skills to assist the parents at a home birth?
- Do you have emergency numbers (the nearest, fastest ambulance service, something other than 911) available?
- Do you know infant CPR (cardio-pulmonary resuscitation)?
- Should you cut the umbilical cord?
- What supplies can you use that are readily available at the home?
- What are the legal liabilities you face if you attend an unexpected home birth?
- What administrative responsibilities will you face if you attend an unexpected home birth? (birth certificates, etc.)
- Who can you call to help if you need it?

The probability of attending an unexpected home birth is remote, but the possibility will always exist. You should consider this carefully if you intend to assist laboring women at home.

Births with a Poor Outcome

When one thinks of assisting at a birth, invariably the wonderful birth with a good outcome comes to mind. But before embarking on this career one needs to give thought to the other births--those with a poor outcome. It is not easy to help families who have a tragic or profoundly disappointing outcome, yet it may be the most important work the labor assistant does. She must decide if she can feel comfortable providing assistance to couples who are grieving. The impact on the family of the loss of a baby or severe illness or disability is great and is even greater if the labor assistant finds the situation so uncomfortable that she withdraws from them emotionally. Quite often the labor assistant is the only person who has contact with the family before, during, and after the loss. Her relationship with the couple might be the most effective and therapeutic relationship of all the family's caregivers.

"In my particular case, she helped the most in her undying devotion to my husband and myself after the tragic birth when I returned home. She helped us through our grief from the beginning, when we discovered the problem, until the death of our baby at three and a half months."

The labor assistant must know strategies which will help the family validate the loss, help make the loss real, and help them adjust to their loss. When it is apparent that the baby has died, the labor assistant should be honest and straightforward with the family. If the baby has not yet been born, she can stress the positive aspects of continuing with their original birth plan. If their dream was to have an unmedicated birth, there is no reason to take that away even if their baby has already been taken from them. The labor assistant should follow the parents' lead in finding the best way to help during such a tragedy.

Once the baby is born, the monitrice or doula should encourage actions which help them accept the infant's death intellectually and emotionally. She should encourage the couple to see and hold their infant, name him or her and call the baby by name, give the baby a bath, and dress him or her. She can help them arrange a religious ceremony if desired by the family. She should encourage the parents to choose the clothes for the baby to be buried in, one of the last parenting tasks they can do for their infant. The labor assistant should find out which funeral homes are sensitive and caring in their handling of the death of an infant. She can help the parents decide whether to have an autopsy and what they want done with the body (burial or cremation). The labor assistant should let the parents know she will be there to support them in their grief, whether they need to talk or to be left alone. Doing these things also helps the labor assistant herself in dealing with the situation.

"When Barbara called and said she hadn't felt the baby move for several days and was going to the hospital to be monitored, I went immediately to her house. I knew the baby was probably dead and wanted to be the one who told her this. It would have broken my heart if someone she didn't even know told her there was no heartbeat."

Labor assistants have demanding jobs. They must care for and nurture their clients, but also be able to deal with conflict effectively. They are on-call twenty four hours a day and must give and give and give though they may be tired from lack of sleep, or stressed from matters unrelated to their clients. They have the pleasure of sharing one of life's most precious moments with couples, but they must be ready to share a couple's greatest grief. Labor assistants may find themselves on emotional rollercoasters because their role requires them to get involved, to care. For some very special women, this career is a life choice.

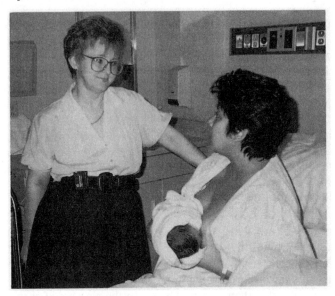

Visiting the mother post-partum to discuss
the birth is one of the roles of the doula.

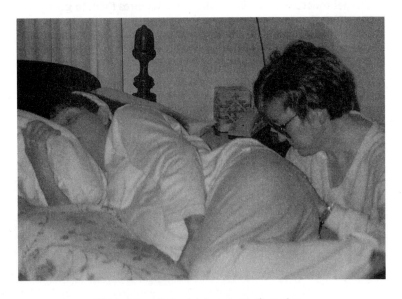

The doula's gentle touch is important to the mother.

4.
Setting up Practice

Many labor assistants initially begin their practice on an informal basis, assisting their friends, relatives, or couples with whom they have become closely involved. While many are content to continue their practice on this informal basis, others go on to develop a professional service. They often do this to gain credibility with other health professionals; to be seen as something other than "the extra person this couple brought along." They want and need to be perceived by nurses, midwives, and doctors see them as part of the health care team.

Most doulas are women and according to the latest statistics gathered by the National Foundation for Women Business Owners, female business owners account for 8 million U. S. businesses and employ one out of four workers, approximately 18.5 million people. You will be joining a group of female-owned business owners and the growth of female-owned businesses outpaces overall business growth by 2-to-1 and is more likely to remain in business than the average firm.

For those starting independent programs, a tough question to ask yourself is whether you are starting this program as a business or a hobby. A private doula service can be run as a hobby with the intent that if you leave, the program will close. Starting small enables one to start as a hobby with the option of growing into a small business. Even with a small business, it helps if you start modestly. Don't bite off more than you can chew.

Several studies done at Harvard Business School have found that business owners attribute 80 percent of their success to acting on intuition. Listen closely when you hear a still, small voice. The voice of the gut is always closer to the truth; gut feelings sometimes tell us about things that we haven't yet consciously identified. You will need more than just intuition though. Starting and running a doula business requires countless hours and tremendous energy. Planning a doula practice begins with determining what the needs of childbearing women are in your community. You'll have greater success if you are filling a need that is easily aroused. In other words, if your program serves a type of hunger in the community, it will be easier to sell the services of a doula. Even though you know what service you can provide, you must also identify the fundamental benefits of the service. Knowing this will help you target your market segment. Do not make the mistake of trying to serve the needs of all segments of your market. Target the type of client you want to serve and focus your service on that market. For instance, do you plan on providing doula services to pregnant teens? Women with low incomes? Women within a certain managed care system? Women who will be delivering at a certain site? Women in a certain geographic area? Women with a certain history (VBAC)? Although your potential clients need to know what services your program will offer, it is infinitely more important for them to know what benefit they will derive from those services. They are much more likely to hire a doula if they know what a doula can do for them.

When planning on starting an independent, private practice, one must also consider the effect of the doula work on your family and children. Being on call 24 hours a day and working unpredictable hours requires that you have support from all those in your intimate personal life. Prior to deciding upon starting a doula business it is helpful if you sit down with your life partner and discuss each family member's needs as well as their expectations of you. Ask yourself, who will supply those needs when you are not there. You need to know if your life partner sees your doula work as a business or as a hobby. Have you thought about being called away during important family holidays or events? It is always better to plan for the worst and have arranged in advance how the situation will be handled, than use denial to cope by thinking these issues will not be a problem. Together, you and your family will set realistic expectations for your doula program. For these reasons, many doulas in private practice start by accepting only a few clients per year and expand their practice as their family adapts to the life of a doula.

As someone interested in offering labor support, you may wish to consider various aspects of the business before venturing into practice. When becoming an entrepreneur and starting a private doula practice you might ask yourself the following questions.

- Am I or can I be a self starter?
- How well do I get along with a variety of personality types?
- Can I make independent decisions?
- Do I have the physical and emotional stamina to run a 24 hour on-call business?
- Am I organized?
- Can I establish realistic time frames?
- Can I tolerate interruptions?
- Can I work with a plan?
- Am I willing to do the research necessary to start a successful business?
- Is my drive strong enough to keep me motivated during "down" times?
- How will this affect my family?

Business information about doula programs can be found in *Doula*

Programs: How to Start and Run a Private or Hospital-Based Program with Success! by Paulina G. Perez and Deaun Thelen.   To avoid re-inventing the wheel, you might want to read it right after attending a doula training.   The book is divided into 14 chapters that cover beginning steps, planning and naming the programs, marketing, third party reimbursement, program development and maintenance, training, self-care for the doula, communication and relationships, troubleshooting, and evaluation.

The authors of the book describe the obstacles to creating change in a hospital. They include politics, fears, conflicts, and hostility, but Perez and Thelen's approach is not confrontational, but strongly positive, constructive, and encouraging.

One of the first steps in setting up a practice as a labor assistant is to decide what kind of care you are going to offer. Be realistic about your skills as well as what can be done in your community.

A written job description is often a good way to help crystallize your thinking about exactly what your role will be. Use the following list to decide which tasks you can or will perform.

Prenatal Services
- Prenatal Counseling Sessions
  - How many? When in the pregnancy?
  - Emotional Assessment
  - Advice on choices (place of birth, childbirth classes, caregiver, baby's healthcare provider, maternity leave, etc.)
  - Review of previous birth and help with emotional healing, if needed.
  - Referrals for services
- Physical Assessment/Prenatal Care
  - Uterine growth
  - Leopold's maneuver
  - Maternal blood pressure checks
  - fetal heart rate determination and interpretation
  - Vaginal examination
  - Non-stress testing
  - Assist client with development of Birth Plan and baby care plan
  - Discussion of role you will play and services you will provide
  - Discussion of doctor's, nurses, and midwife's feelings about your care interfaces with the care they provide
- Recommend reading for client and partner

- Childbirth preparation
- Sibling preparation
- Breastfeeding education
- Home visit prenatally
- Consultation with client's physician or midwife

During Labor
- Out of hospital care
     Home care before going to hospital
     Home birth care
     Early labor care in site close to hospital before going to
          hospital (for those who live far from hospital)
- Maternal physical assessment
     Blood pressure, temperature, reflexes, respiration
     Reading and interpretation of urine test sticks
     Cervical assessment for dilation, effacement and position
          of cervix, station of presenting part
     Nitrazine test for rupture of membranes
     Timing of uterine contractions
- Fetal assessment
     Identification of presentation, position, attitude, variety,
          station, and lie
     Fetal heart tone determination and interpretation
- Emotional support and guidance
- Physical support for comfort and labor progress
- Advice on when to go to hospital or birth center
- Assistance to parents in communicating with other health
  professionals
- Assistance in obtaining cooperation of other providers in
  implementing birth plan
- Consultation with client's physician

During Birth
- Emotional support and guidance
- Physical support
- Application of perineal compresses
- Perineal massage and support
- Assistance with delivery of infant

After Birth
- Review of events of labor and parents' impressions
- Emotional support and guidance
- Physical support

- Assistance with breastfeeding
- Assessment of mother's or baby's physical well-being
- Advice/instruction in baby care

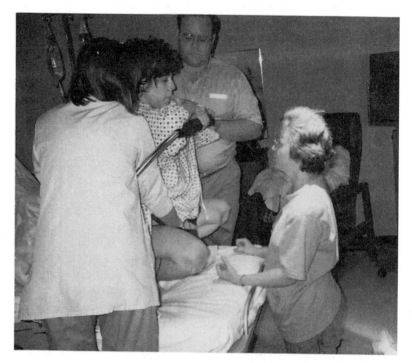

The doula's total focus is on the mother's needs

Doula or Monitrice Services?

The decision whether to provide services that include clinical skills may be a difficult one. Labor assistants who provide physical and emotional support, but no assessment of fetal and maternal well-being, often do so because they feel the other duties would detract from their ability to synchronize themselves with the mother. They want their total focus to be on the mother's needs; to be the only one who does not have to act as a lifeguard and keep an eye out for trouble. Leaving that role to the primary caregiver or nurse frees them to float along with the mother in the sea of emotions and sensations involved with birth. Not having to be aware of fetal or maternal safety allows them to "be one" with the mother, to feel what she is feeling and interpret those feelings to the other people in attendance. These labor assistants generally see themselves as the bridge between the insular, pear-shaped world of the woman in labor and the rest of the birthing team. Others feel that monitoring fetal or maternal well-being blurs the distinction between the labor assistant and the primary care-giver in the parents' minds. Some labor assistants find that obstetricians in their area are more comfortable working with a labor assistant who has a "hands-off policy" and therefore wisely restrict their practice accordingly.

Labor assistants who provide services which involve clinical skills often see those as necessary, especially if they are caring for families outside the hospital setting. Their clients often hire a monitrice because they want skilled care at home, not just emotional support. Clinical skills enable the labor assistant to provide the parents with more detailed information about the condition of mother and baby. This may allow some mothers the confidence they need to labor longer at home ; it allows them greater assurance that labor is progressing and the baby is remaining well. In other instances, the labor assistant can tell the parents that some danger is involved in remaining at home and that transport to the hospital is more appropriate.

Clinical skills might also enable the labor assistant to make recommendations which will allow the mother more effective use of her energy and body during labor. For instance, a vaginal exam to determine the fetus' position and the application of its head to the cervix could be helpful in recommending labor positions. Determination of cervical status might allow the mother to learn to adjust to the sensations of labor. This can be particularly helpful if she interprets contractions to be intense while still early in labor.

Assessment of fetal well-being is important if the parents want to labor at home until late in the first stage. Auscultation of the baby's heart can be performed by a fetoscope or doppler and count the fetal heart rate during a uterine contraction and for 30 seconds after. The American College of Obstetricians and Gynecologists (ACOG) states that the heart rate be monitored intermittently every thirty minutes for low-risk patients in active labor and every 15 minutes in the second stage of labor.(5,6) It is appropriate for someone in attendance to auscultate fetal heart tones every fifteen minutes in active labor. A labor assistant unable to do this task should encourage hospital admission earlier in labor. Professional labor assistants with a nursing background and experience may find it difficult to function only using a portion of their skills and therefore decide to function as a monitrice rather than as a doula.

Establish a Niche for Your Services

Part of becoming a doula or monitrice is determining how the services you provide are different from the services as offered by the hospital staff. This can help avoid "turf struggles" with hospital personnel when you arrive with the birthing couple. Once you find out what is lacking in the hospital care, you can further educate your clients about the need for your particular services. Here are some of the differences.

1) The doula or monitrice has prior knowledge of this couple, and their unique needs. This gives her an advantage over the hospital nurse, who has rarely met the couple. Having developed a trusting relationship prenatally, it is easier for the couple to turn to the labor assistant for recommendations than to the hospital nurse, who is a stranger and an authority figure.

2) A professional labor assistant's loyalties always lie with the birthing couple. Because the couple has hired her, the doula or monitrice is responsible to the couple alone; not to the hospital or physician. The hospital nurse is often put in the difficult position of doing what the hospital or physician or midwife want her to do rather than doing what she feels is best for the birthing couple. It may be much harder for her to suggest all options open to the couple, such as discharge against medical advice, refusing procedures, or trying alternative methods not usually used in the hospital. Her job might be on the line if she speaks out. Many nurses agree with an option suggested by the labor assistant but may be very hesitant to suggest it themselves.

"These couples know me very well before labor even starts. They trust me to tell them what really is happening and not give them a song and dance. They are sure, and rightly so that I have their best interests at heart."

3) Labor assistants and hospital staff also have a different perspective on the amount of time needed to birth. Often hospital personnel come from a very rigid background regarding appropriate lengths of time each phase of labor shall take. The birth assistant often offers the perspective learned in environments other than the hospital. She may realize that time is all the mother needs. She has come to realize that it is perfectly normal for some mothers to push three to four hours to birth their baby, not just for the two hour time limit which is the rule in many hospitals. She is more apt to encourage the mother to take a walk when she seems stuck at six centimeters rather than suggest pain medication or pitocin

augmentation because she has learned from many other walks that movement often results in progress. She also knows that if her manner is loving, unhurried, and accepting, the mother may confide in her about her fear of "letting go." The walk and the talk are often as therapeutic as medication. The labor assistant has time and sustained energy for this individual; the hospital staff may not. These important attributes along with the deeply held belief that women can give birth are often all that is needed to give the mother the faith and willingness to continue.

4) The labor assistant may also be more familiar and comfortable with the use of a variety of positions for labor She not only approves, she encourages the woman to change position and move about. She can assure the mother who feels best laboring while sitting on the toilet that this is perfectly normal and a very good idea, while a nurse with limited experience or inflexible ideas might only encourage her to stay in bed with the monitor attached.

5) When a mother has a midwife, she may assume she does not need the services of the professional labor assistant. This is not necessarily so. Although most midwives provide excellent support, they too represent varied philosophies. In addition, some are expected to attend more than one laboring woman at a time, to perform other clinical tasks, or to comply with institutional ideas. If problems arise, the midwife has to concern herself primarily with clinical management and may find it difficult to manage the problem and provide adequate emotional support simultaneously. Midwives who have hospital based practices rarely go to the couple's home in early labor; the labor assistant is able to help this couple avoid early hospitalization just as she would with a physician caregiver. Even in the case of home births it is often important to have another person there whose sole responsibility is to support the mother.

"I work as a labor assistant mainly at home births and find that often I am the only one who doesn't have to worry in the way that the primary caregiver does. She must act as a lifeguard and keep an eye out for trouble. I am there simply to be with the mother and interpret what she is feeling or what she needs to others."

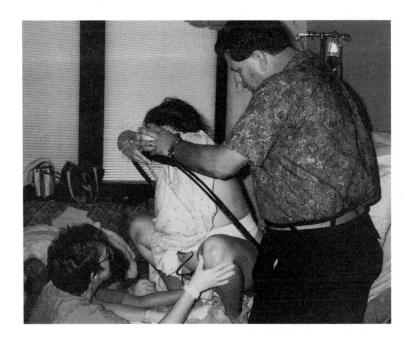

When a labor assistant recommends a variety of
labor positions she must be pretty flexible herself.

Learning As You Go

Some labor assistants see their role as a continuum, beginning with
emotional support, and growing as they learn additional skills. They
must let their clients know their limitations and that they are learning
new skills. Couples should be given a choice when the novice monitrice
wishes to practice new skills such as vaginal exams, fetal heart tones,
etc. Once the client is in the hospital, those tasks are performed by the
nursing staff, while the labor assistant continues with emotional and
physical support.

Marketing and Public Relations

Much of a doula or monitrice's business is built on referrals therefore
it is important to know referral techniques to continue bringing in new
clients. This is especially true in a private practice where the marketing

budget is often very small. Doulas and monitrices excel at building long-term relationships. This trait will be of great benefit when trying to build a practice.   Building strong, lasting relationships with clients increases repeat business as well as referrals. One-time clients become repeat clients when they know that the doula or monitrice cares about them and their needs.

To encourage current or past clients to refer others to your business, always remind them that you are looking for new business.   It is amazing how well this simple tip works in generating referrals.

A marketing plan should be used as a map to generate more business; it is a set of steps that will help you achieve the goals you have set. Without a well thought out marketing plan, you will waste both time and money. This plan does not have to be an extensive one; it can be a page or two. You may have two marketing plans- one for short term goals and one for long term goals. The short term plan may include things such as getting publicity in local papers and easily fits into the long term plan. Your long term marketing plan which is built on your goals, will tell who you are, what you do, why you do it and how to promote your business long range. The long term plan will help you to project into the future and look at what could happen to the program under various situations.   This is especially important with all the changes that are constantly occurring within the health care field as a whole.

Unlike many other cultures, the role of the doula is new in this culture. Be patient when trying to educate others about professional labor assistants. For doulas and monitrices in private practice, person to person and print media seem to be the most affordable options. When telling others about the role of the professional labor assistant, translate objections into questions so that your answers do not sound defensive. As soon as you hear the objection, rephrase it mentally to yourself as a question. Turn the objections into reasons to hire a doula. Before you answer an objection, show empathy and understanding for your client or interviewer by agreeing with them on some point.   You have now cushioned your statement with an empathy statement. The person you are talking to needs to know that they have been heard and are understood. Do not be afraid to admit your limitations.

Doulas and monitrices can benefit from having a web page. First, decide what message to deliver on the web page. When writing the page, be concise and state your message clearly. Create a personal feeling with a short bio or pictures. Make sure your buttons look like buttons. If your site includes more than one page, identify each page and include a link back to your home page.   Don't include too many complicated graphics as people get frustrated waiting for them to load and may click off your site.   Besides your e-mail address, include your mailing address, phone and FAX numbers.

Network with other businesses whose clients are likely to need your services or whose services your clients need.   These might include postpartum doula services, baby stores, lactation consultants, maternity stores, childbirth educators, birth centers, midwives, and physicians. When setting up your practice you might want to set up appointments with local midwives and physicians to explain your services. You can leave business cards or brochures explaining your services with them to distribute to their clients. Visit the childbirth educators in your community, and offer to come to their classes to explain your services and why they are valuable to the family. Leave promotional material in baby stores, healthfood stores, bookstores, and offices of pediatricians, family practitioners, chiropractors and massage therapists. Attend La Leche League meetings to discuss the value of professional labor support.   Offer to teach a class at your local birth center on labor support. A doula in private practice in New Jersey has used a very novel way to advertise her services. She goes to the sales office of new home developments and tells them about her business and that it is beneficial information for new families moving into their homes. She leaves them a business card holder with her cards in it and then replenishes it regularly. Doulas who are just starting an independent practice might also want to call local birth centers and other doulas in the area and let them know that they are willing to take clients who cannot afford a doula as a way to gain experience. Let your local ICAN or VBAC support group know of your services; become involved with their group. Mention the benefits of professional labor support in childbirth classes that you teach, although you must be careful not to make the classes simply an advertising vehicle.

"I have not been promoting myself as assertively as when my services were free. I know I'm worth the fee but part of me hangs back from promoting myself too strongly in my classes for fear people may interpret that I'm using my $50 classes as an advertising vehicle for my $125 labor support services."

Solo or Partnership?

Decide if you will practice alone, in a partnership or as part of a group. If you practice alone be aware that you will still need someone who can back you up in times of other obligations, illness, emergencies or when you have two women laboring at the same time. If you are part of a partnership or group be sure it is clear when you are on call and establish procedures for time off.

How will your clients reach you? If you provide only occasional labor support, frequent phone contact is often all that is needed. A calendar indicating how and where to reach you every day might also be helpful. If you have a rather busy service a beeper which can be leased or purchased can solve the problem of multiple phone calls to your clients regarding your location. There are many types of pagers--tone pagers, digital pagers, pagers that vibrate to alert you of a call. Research all types, charges, etc. See "Paging Systems" in the yellow pages. An answering service that knows your location is another option.

Decide if you will charge for your services. If you choose not to charge a fee, will you ask for a donation or reimbursement for expenses (babysitting, transportation, parking, food)? If you decide to charge a fee, what will it be? A flat fee? An hourly rate? A flat fee for a certain number of hours combined with an hourly rate thereafter? Will you accept a sliding scale fee structure? Will you barter for your services? Will you require a deposit when a client books your services? Do you expect the fee to be paid in advance? At the time of the birth? After the birth? Will you accept a payment schedule? Will you and are you eligible to accept insurance reimbursement? If you are a registered nurse, your services may be covered as private duty nursing or home health monitoring. A physician's or midwife's order is usually required for third party reimbursement. Labor assistant's fees range widely depending on the assistant's training and background and the area of the country in which she práctices. Generally, the fees of labor assistants in North America range between gratis and $1000, with $300-$400 an average fee. Monitrices with additional clinical skills usually charge more for their services with $600-$1,000 being an average fee.

Fees are collected in a variety of ways. Some practitioners charge a deposit that is payable on the first visit and the remainder at the time of service. Some have the entire fee due payable at approximately 36 weeks into the pregnancy while others offer the client the option of paying by credit card. In order to receive credit card payments, the doula or monitrice must have established credit card services with banks or a credit card service agency.

If you will be receiving third party reimbursement, it will be helpful for you to be familiar with diagnosis and procedure codes. They can be found in ICD-9-CM Codebooks. These books are used by medical offices and hospitals. You might consider purchasing one for your personal use. The use of diagnosis and procedure codes speeds up the reimbursement process.

Most often the client pays you directly, and you give her a bill showing that she has paid. She submits that for reimbursement. Be sure your bill includes the following information: your name, address, credentials and professional license number; date of the bill; name and address of the client; description of services provided; the date you provided the services; the diagnosis or diagnoses; the fee; amount paid; and the name of the provider who ordered the services. Insurance forms and other labor assistant supplies are available from Cutting Edge Press. Some insurers request a copy of the written order or request letter from the provider, and a copy of your nursing notes to verify the services provided.

Record Keeping

In business, ask yourself how will you use this record and how important the information is? The importance in keeping good records cannot be over emphasized. These records must be able to substantiate your tax returns under both federal and state which include both income tax and Social Security. They will also be needed for professional liability and other professional reasons.

Paperwork is usually the least favorite part of the professional labor assistant's job, but it is essential. You can custom design your own forms or purchase printed forms. *Labor Support Forms: A Guide to Doula Charting* by Cheri Grant includes the following forms that are of help to the doula or monitrice: prenatal forms, intrapartum forms, postpartum forms, insurance forms, doula records, doula brochures, income and expense forms. The author allows individuals to adapt the form for their personal use. These forms as well as many other doula-related items may be purchased from Cutting Edge Press, a professional labor assistant owned business (802/635-2142 or http://www.childbirth.org/CEP.html).

It is often helpful to develop a contract for use in your practice. This may be as simple as a form that lists what the professional labor assistant will and will not do, the obligations of both the labor assistant and the client, the services the doula or monitrice will provide and provisions for payment with an area for the labor assistant, the client and her partner to sign. This type form is included in *Labor Support Forms: A Guide to Doula Charting* by Cheri Grant, RN

Professional Organizations for the Professional Labor Assistant

Professional labor assistants often join a professional organization like DONA, ICEA, ALACE, Childbirth Enhancement Foundation, and Lamaze International. Some of these organizations train and certify others and others only train them but do not certify them. These organizations have mission statements and standards of practice, a code of ethics under which the professional labor assistant will practice. Consult the above groups for their standards of practice and code of ethics.   Ethical considerations include rules of conduct, provision for backup, responsibility to clients, colleagues, other health care workers and the profession as a whole.   Competency is an important issue as there is no licensure to assure this.

Topics for Doula Training Course
The following topics are usually covered in a doula training course.
Definition of professional labor assistants/doulas/monitrices
Code of Ethics
Standards of Practice
Care Protocol and Procedures
Introduction to labor support
Working with other support people
A Woman's birth experience and her life
Additional recommended reading
Terminology
Premature labor
Early Labor
Active labor
Transition
Second stage of labor
Third stage of labor
Apgar scoring
Cervical effacement and dilatation
Electronic fetal monitoring
Physiology of pain
Pain management
Relaxation techniques
Assessing relaxation
Breathing techniques
Assessment of coping skills
Support skills for labor and birth
Physical and emotional comfort measures
Back pain in labor
Physiological effects of heat and cold
Panic routine
Comfort positions for labor
Role play labor situations and comfort/support techniques
Supplies for your birth bag
Drugs and childbirth
Medications that relieve pain during childbirth
Epidural anesthesia
Spinal anesthesia

Fetal presentations
IV's
Induction or augmented labors
Episiotomy
Forceps-assisted births
Vacuum-assisted births
Complications
AIDS precautions
Triple screen test
The Doula and Cesarean section
VBAC
Special Issues
 Birth in other cultures
 Teen pregnancy
 Infant death and grief issues
Breastfeeding
Bottle-feeding
Postpartum Adjustment
Postpartum Emotions and Postpartum Mood Reactions
Siblings and the newborn
Newborn characteristics
Newborn exam
Postpartum follow-up protocol
Patient care coordination
Social work services
Community resources
Pregnant patient Bill of Rights/Responsibilities
Communication skills
Reflective listening skills
Team building
Resolving conflicts
Post Test
Doula Forms
 Scheduling
 Birth story
Doula self care
Professional Labor Assistant Organizations
 DONA
 ALACE
 ICEA
 Childbirth Enhancement Foundation
A complete labor assistant training syllabus can be obtained from
Cutting Edge Press. See Resources at the end of this book for more

information on how to contact the company.

Professional Attire

Professional labor assistants often choose scrubs of their own choice which are separate from hospital attire and identify them as professionals. The advantage of this is the ability to have a set or two of clothes that are for work only and are always clean and ready to wear. Another option for the PLA is to wear a scrub jacket over her street clothes. Although some professional labor assistants feel that wearing any hospital type attire (scrubs, jackets, etc.) might make them be seen as "one of the hospital," others find that the potential for hospital personnel seeing them in a more professional manner is ultimately of greater benefit to the laboring mother. It is often amazing how something so simple creates such a dramatic change in how hospital personnel treat the doula or monitrice and thus enables her to be of more help to the laboring woman.

Disease Protection

The doula or monitrice should comply with OSHA guidelines for disease protection. Human Immunodeficiency Virus (HIV) and Hepatitis B (HBV) precautions should be followed by all those involved directly with patient care, including professional labor assistants. Breaks in the skin and mucous membranes are potential entry points for both viruses, therefore close attention must be taken to avoid contact with bodily fluids. Barrier protections such as gloves, gowns, masks and goggles may be used to prevent the caregiver from exposure. The clothing the doula wears should either be washable (shoes included) or disposable. Avoid contact with uncapped needles or sharp instruments. The doula and monitrice should wear gloves when in contact with body fluids as in instances of changing bed linen, patient gowns, and towels, when the mother has ruptured membranes, when she starts pushing, applying compresses to the perineum or handling the unbathed newborn. Hospitals now provide gloves in all patient rooms for use by hospital personnel, including doulas and monitrices.

Initial Contact and Interview

The ability to meet one's doula before actually going into labor can help to give the woman a greater sense of peace and well being. This may also help a woman who is feeling apprehensive about her impending labor to feel more safe and in control. After speaking briefly with couples who call to inquire about your services, you might offer to send them written material as a follow-up. This material could include your promotional brochure, business card, articles describing the value of labor support (1,2,3,4), letters of reference from former clients and a list of questions to ask of any labor support professional they might potentially hire. You might also offer to set up a time for them to come in to interview you at length regarding your services. See page 22, "Interview Questions," for ideas on what to discuss at this initial meeting.

Prenatal Interview

You will need the following information about your client.

Client's Name:_____
Partner's Name:_____
Address:_____
Home Phone:_____Pager:_____
Her Work #_____His Work #:_____
OB/Midwife:_____phone:_____
Hospital:_____ _phone:_____
Pediatrician:_____ ___phone:_____
Due Date:_____Client's Birth date:_____

I.   Health History

1. Please describe your health in general (pre-pregnancy)
2. Blood Type
3. Drug allergies or reactions
4. Any chronic illnesses
5. List any medications you take regularly
6. List any surgeries along with date of treatment
7. List any infertility treatments along with date of procedures
8. List any emotional disorders along with date of onset & types of treatment
9. Do you have any concerns about your well-being?

Charting

Accurately documenting what happens in the labor and birth is extremely important for both quality of care and medical-legal reasons. The charting of a monitrice is often more detailed than a doula's as her care comprises emotional support, physical support and clinical observations.   Monitrices' charts often resemble nursing notes or midwifery charting. Charting by doulas usually contain a running log about maternal activity and positions, statistics (exams and procedures) and personal notations (how mother and partner interact, client reactions, etc.) Doula Felicia Roche has compiled a doula charting system that contains the following sheets: client contact sheet, prenatal interview notes, contract/agreement, receipt for payment, prenatal interview, *Your Birth Plan and Your Birth* by Paulina Perez, and labor notes. *Labor Support Forms: A Guide to Doula Charting* by Cheri Grant contains a comprehensive set of forms for a labor support business. The author has given the reader the right to copy the forms. She only asks that the professional labor assistant using the forms, give the author credit by retaining the line across the bottom of each form. Both the doula charting system and *Labor Support Forms* and other labor support supplies are available through Cutting Edge Press. Doulas of North America (DONA) has a birth record sheet that contains the following information: client profile, site of birth, type of room, type of primary care provider, gestation at delivery, time labor contractions began, dilatation/effacement/station when admitted to the hospital, spontaneous rupture of membranes, presence of meconium, labor progression, use of medical interventions and procedures, length of first, second and third stages, time doula arrived and departed, and information about the baby (time of birth, sex, weight, length, Apgars, transfer to NICU, resuscitative efforts).

Restrictions in Practice

If you restrict your practice in any way, be honest with prospective clients about your reasons for those decisions. Some labor assistants will work in any setting. Others feel uncomfortable providing labor support for women giving birth outside of the hospital (home or birth center). Still others prefer to work in settings outside the hospital.

"I started to burn out working with couples in the hospital and felt that I couldn't give them my best so I began to focus my practice more on home births."

Some labor assistants believe that if they limit where and with whom they will work, they are limiting choices available to the birthing couple. They feel they are there to enhance the birth, not put restrictions on it. Others prefer to work in specific hospitals, but will go wherever the client has chosen. If they can still function effectively in a less supportive environment, the value to the couple is highly beneficial. They realize that the worse the environment, the more the couple needs their support. They do try to make the couple aware of the reality of and potential risks of birthing in such an unfavorable environment. Some labor assistants have found, usually through trial and error, that the environment at particular hospitals is not at all conducive to a natural birth. They choose not to work in hospitals where the attitude is one of antagonism and hostility, with strict and unbending rules.

"One hospital is too hard on my nerves. My experiences there have left me so angry at how the mother was treated that I decided no amount of money could compensate me for attending births there."

Hospital rules may restrict your practice. Some hospitals limit the people who may be in attendance at labor and/or birth. They may state that no third party may be present or that only one person is able to attend the mother. In that case, a labor assistant would be able to attend a birth only if the father is not there. A hospital might allow a labor assistant only if she is on the hospital staff. Some hospitals will allow the presence of the labor assistant if the birth occurs in a birthing room or LDR room but may refuse to allow the labor assistant to attend if the birth occurs in the delivery room or surgery suite. Sometimes these "rules" are really only customs which can be challenged by parents working with their labor assistants. Labor assistants should be willing to work with couples who want to change such "rules."

Labor assistants may also restrict their practice by working only with particular caregivers--those who welcome them and value their contributions. Some physicians are unsupportive of natural birth no matter who is in attendance or what the outcome. Some physicians "talk a good story" but deliver standard, conventional care. Through experience, labor assistants learn which physicians have abnormally high cesarean rates. Some physicians refuse to work with professional labor assistants or they allow them to be present but refuse to see them as health care professionals. Others begrudgingly allow the presence of the labor assistant but treat her as a "fifth wheel." With such a lack of acceptance, a labor assistant might find that her presence is a detriment to the client. She may have to refuse to work in that environment. Some labor assistants restrict their practice to a particular type of client, for example, VBAC clients, pregnant teens, or racial or ethnic minorities.

"I refuse to work in certain hospitals and with certain physicians because I have seen my clients "punished" for being assertive and for hiring extra support."

The Postpartum Component

A comprehensive postpartum follow up visit is done following the birth experience. This is usually done approximately two weeks following the birth although that may vary depending upon the mother's needs. These visits may often coincide with their postpartum follow up visit with their primary caregiver. The aim of the postpartum visit by the professional labor assistant is not only to bring closure to the relationship but to leave the mother with a feeling of accomplishment and give the labor assistant feedback about her services. The doula or monitrice might want to ask the following feedback questions of both the mother and her partner.

1. Is there anything you would change about the labor and birth?
2. Were you as involved in the birth as you wanted to be?
3. How did having a professional labor assistant benefit you?
4. As the partner, was there any time you felt excluded by the presence of a labor assistant?
5. What did the labor assistant do during the labor and birth that was most helpful to you as the father? Mother?
6. Was there anything that you did not like that the labor assistant did? Be specific.
7. How do you feel about the amount of time the labor assistant spent with you? Too little? More than needed? Just right?
8. What were your reasons for hiring a labor assistant? Would you hire a labor assistant again for subsequent births? Would you recommend this service to others?
9. What did the labor assistant do during the pregnancy and postpartum that was most helpful to you as the mother? Father?
10. What did you feel was the most important part of having a professional labor assistant?

The labor assistant should review her birth log prior to the postpartum follow-up meeting to refresh her memory of the birth.   Information gained during the postpartum follow up visit should be documented and kept as part of the client's record. Giving the mother a written copy of her birth story is not only appreciated by the mother at this time, but often remains a permanent part of the child's baby book. It can also be just that little extra special touch that sets your service apart from others. This birth story, written by the doula or monitrice, recaps the special moments of birth and often plays a part in the overall satisfaction the mother feels about her birth experience. The birth story can be written as a congratulatory letter to the mother, a letter from the baby, or a letter from the professional labor assistant about the events of the day. Many professional labor assistants bring a closure gift to the postpartum visit. Examples of these simple gifts are a hand-painted baby tee shirt, knitted newborn hat, breastfeeding or baby care book, potpourri for the mom, pictures from the birth, picture frame with a birth photo, herbal bath salts, or a scrap book for the mother starting with the headlines from the newspaper published on the day of her baby's birth. Let your creativity run wild here as you select a gift. This small gift is often a token of the bond formed between the laboring woman and her professional birth assistant. Often on your final postnatal meeting, you might ask the new parents if you can give their name as a reference to prospective clients.

Comfort Measures and Labor Support Strategies
When assessing labor pain consider the following:
   Remember "When in doubt check it out."
   Ask the mother the following questions.
   What's going through your mind?
   Is there something you are afraid of?
   What do you think will help?
   What's wrong?
   Is there something that you are frightened of?
   Tell me how you feel.
   Encourage the mother to empty her bladder hourly.
   Make sure the mother remains well hydrated.
   Encourage the mother to relax her voluntary muscles in her buttocks,
   thighs, abdomen and pelvic floor.

Remind the mother to ambulate and change positions often so that her baby will be in the optimal fetal position or birth. Changes in the mother's position often has beneficial effects on the pelvic bones, contractions, and oxygen supply to the fetus. The following lists many of the different possible changes in position that can help the mother during birth.

standing	leaning	rocking
swaying	side-lying	sitting
lunge	slow-dancing	dangle
squat	stomp-squat	supported squat
kneeling	hands and knees	sitting on birth ball
hands and knees over birth ball		

The book *Birth Balls: Use of Physical Therapy Balls in Maternity Care* by Paulina G.Perez, RN covers the topic of "birth balls." The physical therapy ball has been in use for about 40 years and professional labor assistants Polly Perez, RN and Penny Simkin, PT began using the "birth ball" to instruct childbirth education students, nurses, midwives, physicians, and professional labor assistants about ten years ago. This versatile ball has a myriad of uses in obstetrics which include the mother staying fit and facilitating labor. The use of the "birth ball" elicits spontaneous non-habituating movement and is a requisite tool for the doula, monitrice, nurse and midwife.

Trust in the professional labor assistant is a prominent aspect of labor support. This involves taking time to explore issues with the pregnant woman. The doula or monitrice helps keep the atmosphere in the birth room   intimate as the entrance of people unknown to the laboring woman and abrupt movements can cause the flight-or-fight mechanism and inhibit labor progress. The professional labor assistant has many "tricks of the trade" to offer the laboring woman.   Her continuous undivided attention is vital to the laboring woman. Attending immediately to pain lets the pregnant woman know that the doula or monitrice will be there to comfort her and suggest many coping strategies for mediating pain.   Painful stimuli coming from pain receptors can be reduced by movement and position.[7]   Increasing the transmission of innocuous impulses so that they compete with painful impulses at the level of the dorsal horn are accomplished by massage, acupressure, hydrotherapy and heat and cold.   Techniques like relaxation, visualization, music therapy and hypnosis help by controlling somatic and autonomic activity.   Music is a helpful labor support strategy. Because music is nonverbal, it can move through the auditory cortex directly to the center of emotional responses in the limbic system, causing relaxation, or feelings of well-being and joy.[8]   It can also enhance rhythmic movement or breathing.   Familiar and well-loved music increases endorphin production, which relieves pain by acting on specific receptors in the brain.   Music also helps establish an inviting environment and can serve as a pleasing distraction from the stress or pain of labor. Modifying the mother's reactions to pain by focusing her attention elsewhere, using rituals, using patterned breathing and guided imagery can also be helpful.

The labor support strategies used by the professional labor assistant include heat, cold, hydrotherapy, acupressure, counterpressure, double hip squeeze, knee press, roving body check, touch, relaxation techniques, use of ritual, reflexology, abdominal stroking, hand massage, dangle, body massage, abdominal lift , slow dancing, pelvic rocking, the "birth ball," panic routine, stomp-squat, lap squat, towel pull and maternal positions like walking, stair climbing, sitting, kneeling, hands and knees, swaying, squatting, and asymmetrical upright positions.   Consider keeping a set of Labor Support Cards or a copy of *The Nurturing Touch at Birth* in your birth bag when you are in a "What do I do now situation."

The labor assistant should also be familiar with information about medications to ameliorate pain like analgesics, anesthetics, and intracutaneous injections of sterile water so that she can provide the pregnant couple information to make a informed choice.   Analgesics like Demerol, Nubain, Stadol, Morphine and Talwin are used to reduce, abolish or alter the mother's perception of pain.   They promote relaxation between contractions. They are most frequently administered during the active phase of labor or for post partum pain relief after a cesarean section. The side effects of these drugs to the mother can be dizziness, nausea, and decreased blood pressure. The side effects of these drugs to the baby can be changes in fetal heart rate pattern, depression of respiration and infant behavior responses postpartum. The regional anesthetics like epidural, spinal, pudendal, and local are given by injection and produce loss of sensation in a particular region of the body supplied by the nerves blocked. Epidural side effects to the mother include decrease in blood pressure, inability to void, decrease in contractions, inhibition of bearing-down reflex, increased need for forceps or vacuum, post partum headache, and, infrequently, paralysis. Epidural side effects to the baby include changes if fetal heart rate pattern (notably bradycardia) and alteration in neurological behavior after birth (poor muscle tone, poor sucking response, etc.). The baby can also be indirectly affected by the maternal response to the anesthetics. Intracutaneous injections of sterile water may act as a long segmental acupuncture which works though at lease two mechanisms: stimulation of fast conducting A fibers which affect interneurones in the substantia gelatinosa, producing pain inhibition or by raising the endorphin levels in the spinal fluid. General anesthetics are usually inhaled in gaseous form and produce loss of consciousness. The side effects of general anesthesia to the mother are respiratory depression, decrease in blood pressure, change in heart rate and increase in incidence of postpartum hemorrhage. The side effects to the baby may include respiratory depression, poor muscle tone and lower Apgar scores.

During the pushing phase the professional labor assistant can encourage the mother by saying the following things:

*Listen to your body.

*Push as your body tells you.

*Drop your shoulders and jaw.

      A relaxed mouth helps keep the vagina relaxed.

*Open your eyes and watch your baby come out.

*Reach down and feel your baby.

*Use the time in between contractions to get your energy back. See the energy flowing back into your body.

*Let your baby out slowly.

*Feel how close your baby is to being born.

*The burning sensation is your body's way of saying "Slow down, easy now."

*Reach down and bring your baby up to yourself.

*Talk to your baby.

*Dry your baby off.

Your Birth Bag

Since labor assistants work all hours, it's a good idea to have all your equipment in one bag that is readily available when you get that middle-of-the-night call. The list below should give you some ideas. If you are providing labor support only, you will need just a few of the items (those indicated with an asterisk). If you are providing full scope homecare, consider carrying all the items listed below:

small pelvic model with baby *
clock with second hand *
client records *
any reference book you feel you might need
  (i.e.: *Nurturing Touch at Birth, Special Women*)*
client file *
Labor Support Cards *
scrub jacket or sweater *
herbal tea bags/ loose tea *
honey sticks (about 1TB)*
rice hot sock *
comfort wrap *
lip balm *
labeled (PLA phone #) extra lip balm *
mini-massagers *
Happy Massager *
silica gel cold packs *
rolling pin *
hand held fan *
slipper socks *
hand held mirror *
disposable camera/ film *
tape recorder and audio tapes *
CD or music tapes *
written visualizations *
stress squeeze ball *
combs for acupressure *
extra AA batteries *
note pad and extra pens *
flexible drinking straws *
inflatable tub pillow *
foot lotion *
reusable gel hot/cold packs *
visualization cards from Childbirth Kit *
"tug-of-war" dog pull toy*
1 foot section of pool noodle *

eye pillow *
personal items for PLA *
soapless hand cleaner *
toothbrush and toothpaste *
mouthwash *
breath mints or gum *
Tylenol or Excedrin *
deodorant *
comb/brush and hairspray *
rubber bands *
complete set of clean comfortable work clothes/
scrub clothes *
business cards *
masking tape for notes--tape a piece down the leg of your pants for
quick notes *
ID badge *
throw away catalogs or short book*
garden knee pads *
contact lens case *
healthy "snack" items *
microwaveable lunch *
vending machine change *
doppler with conduction gel and/or fetoscope
sphygmomanometer
stethoscope
nitrazine paper
sterile exam gloves
non-sterile exam gloves
non-latex gloves
water soluble lubricant, preferably sterile
povidone-iodine solution
enema bag
thermometer
tape measure
little cotton pads for aromatherapy
birthing stool
disposable underpads for bed
infant hat
urine test strips
peri bottle

Some labor assistants also pack an "emergency bag" in case they must
assist at an unplanned home birth.

cord clamps
hemostat
scissors
newborn hat
plastic backed sheet
maternity napkins
gauze pads
herbal sitz bath materials
resuscitation equipment

Many of the clinical items are readily available from midwifery supply houses. Check the yellow pages in your area or see "Resources" in this book for more information.   Three types of birth bags (starter, advanced and professional) for labor assistants are available from Cutting Edge Press. Call (802) 635-2142 for further information.

It is important that you remain well nourished and hydrated during labor so you will stay in top form to help the laboring couple. Eat what you need to keep your energy level high. Protein foods (cheese, yogurt, and hard boiled eggs) complex carbohydrates (fruit, whole grain breads and crackers) and fruit juices or sparkling water are healthier than coffee and candy bars. Pack some of these items with you when you leave to join your clients at home or at the hospital, or ask your clients to pack them for you. Hospitals are notorious for having bad food. Sometimes,   especially in the middle of the night, the only food available is from a vending machine.

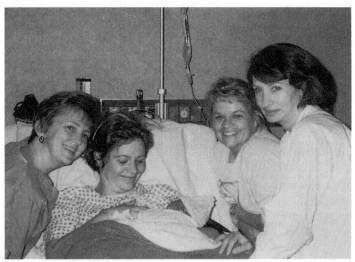

Three labor assistants, who work together, celebrate this baby's birth.

Professional Image

Communicating with other health professionals is another important aspect of setting up your practice. Think of yourself as a professional. This is the first step toward communicating effectively with other members of the health care team. Remember that a professional will act from a solid foundation of informed judgment, educated skill, and a trained instinct, rather than simply react. Your actions are a reflection not only of yourself as an individual, but of your profession as a whole. If you have trouble thinking of yourself as a professional, repeat to yourself, "I am a professional" until you believe it. The very act of repeating this phrase has great power. When you believe that you are professional, you will act in a professional way. That in itself will encourage others to see you in a different light. Once they realize that you see yourself as a professional, their actions toward you may change.

No doula or monitrice can afford to alienate other clinicians. This is why the labor assistant needs to understand the nursing and medical staff roles as well as hospital politics. The presence of the doula or monitrice does not mean that the other clinician's relationships with the laboring woman can no longer take on an emotional component. The labor assistant often acts as a bridge among the others in on the maternity care team. These topics will be covered in more depth in chapter ten.

"I am often thought of by the staff as a friend who wants to see a birth until they notice that I chart. One nurse who initially seemed offended and acted hostile when she noted me charting was more open and accepting at a later birth. She even shared with me a little at this later birth."

References:

[1] "Labor Support," *C-SEC Newsletter*, C-SEC, Inc.,Framingham, MA.

[2] "Labor," J.H. Kennell, in *Birth, Interaction, and Attachment*, Johnson and Johnson, 1982, Silkman, NJ.

[3] "Let your couples know about the role of the professional labor assistant," Paulina Perez, *International Journal of Childbirth Education,* May 1989.

[4] "Birth Assistant: New Ally for Parents-to-Be," Beth Shearer, *Childbirth Educator,* Spring 1989.

[5] "Fetal heart rate patterns: Monitoring, Interpretation, and management, American College of Obstetrician Technical Bulletin No 209, Washington, DC, 1995

[6.] "Standards and guidelines for professional nursing practice in the care of women and newborns," Association of Women's Health, Obstetrics and Neonatal Nurses, Washington, DC, 1998.

[7.] "Nursing, maternal postures, and fetal position," Andrews, C, & Andrews, E., *Nurs Res*, 32(6), 336, 1983.

[8.] "Music and Sound in the Healing Arts," Beaulieu, J, Station Hill Tarrytown, NY, 1987.

5.
Advocacy, Communication, and Community Image

There are at least three components of the labor assistant's role: first, are the personal qualities of kindness, patience, commitment, and interest in the birth process; second, are the practical, hands-on skills of labor support and care; third, are the ability and willingness to advocate for the woman in a maternity care system that is sometimes unresponsive and rigid. This last--the role of patient advocate--is in some ways the most difficult because it implies that conflict may exist between caregiver and client. If so, the woman and her partner, who are vulnerable, stressed, and lacking in knowledge, need someone to help them in their attempt to use alternatives they desire, safely and appropriately.

The labor assistant is hired or invited by the woman or couple not only because of her understanding of laboring and laboring woman but also because of her specialized knowledge about maternity care. She represents the clients' wishes and needs to other health care professionals. She is usually not employed by a physician, a midwife, or hospital, and thus has no allegiance to anyone but her clients. If she is employed by a caregiver, she has a potential conflict of interest if her client and the caregiver have disagreements. She will need to establish a clear understanding with both as to her primary advocacy.   Advocacy does not mean taking over for the woman or couple and making decisions for them or controlling them; it is helping women or couples help themselves by providing them with information and advice. It is important that the doula and monitrice understand the difference in being responsible to others and being responsible for others as she is responsible to her clients but not responsible for them.

When you feel responsible *to* others...

> You show empathy, encourage, share, confront, level, are sensitive, listen.
>
> You feel relaxed, free, aware, high self-esteem.
>
> You are concerned with relating person to person, feelings, and the person.
>
> You are a helper/guide.
>
> You expect the person to be responsible for themselves and their actions.
>
> You can trust and let go.

When you feel responsible *for* others...

> You fix, protect, rescue, control, carry their feelings, don't listen.
>
> You feel tired, anxious, fearful, liable.
>
> You are concerned with the solution, answers, circumstances, being right, details.
>
> You are a manipulator.
>
> You expect the person to live up to your expectations.

The professional labor assistant makes sure her clients are aware of their options so they can make informed choices.

"I wanted to be able to ask questions of someone other than the doctor."

She makes sure the staff sees and respects the woman's or couple's birth plan. She does not   reinforce the feelings of vulnerability, helplessness and dependency that often surface during hospitalization. Instead she supports the parent's efforts towards independence; she inspires them to be advocates for themselves. She encourages them to seek individual solutions to their problems. Advocacy means forming a partnership with the parents with mutual sharing of information, tasks, and efforts.

"We wanted someone who could be a spokesperson yet know when the doctor and hospital staff were justified in saying that the procedures were necessary."

The labor assistant also has a knowledge of the political side of the maternity care system, and therefore   may be more skilled than her clients in negotiating within that system.

"She really knew how to finesse the system for our benefit."

The labor assistant helps the woman or couple establish goals and priorities before labor and accomplish them by focusing their attention during labor on their vision for the birth they want. The mother and her partner must be willing to work hard to achieve her goal. It does no good for the labor assistant to want things for the woman if the woman is not willing to do the intense physical and emotional work necessary to birth.

The Labor Assistant as Change Agent

Our values and beliefs light the way for us as we act as change agents in the maternity care system. We are system thinkers and believe that everything is connected. We believe that the power of large organizations is derived from its members and that a healthy environment maintains its diversity. We believe that we are responsible for the consequences of our actions. We believe that people are the changers in organizations.

If we are to be change agents we need the following skills: management, personal learning, coaching, stress tolerance, and positive political skills. We need to be calculated risk-takers, a lovers of change, open minded, ethical, persistent, imaginative, empathetic, inspiring and empowering.

The labor assistant needs to be known as someone who does a top-notch job. Other health professionals as well as potential clients must know that she is honest and honorable and will help provide safe passage for those in her care. She must develop a reputation for avoiding unnecessary risks, for solving problems quickly, and for referring clients to others when appropriate.

Besides providing safe care, the labor assistant must also understand the political or social context of her role. Her role often identifies her as a leader in the childbearing community. She must know how to influence both individual and group behavior. Her role involves being a change agent and her success may depend on influencing others to work toward change in maternity care--to better meet the needs of expectant women and their families.

The labor assistant must acknowledge and take responsibility for her part in the maternity care system, remembering that problems or difficulties are not always someone else's fault. Labor assistants often see themselves as powerless, continually blaming others for what is happening to mothers and their babies. Power is simply the ability to affect something, and professional labor assistants certainly do affect the lives of those in their care as well as the lives of those other health care professionals with whom they work.

A strong self image and responsible nature are integral components of a change agent. The labor assistant must perceive her contribution as valuable to the maternity care system as a whole. She must look closely at her beliefs about maternity care. What truly is her philosophy of maternity care? Is she willing to make this philosophy public? What are her personal beliefs and values? Do her own interests take precedence over the interests of childbearing families? She often must put the needs of those her clients before herself or her family. She must keep asking herself why she is a labor assistant. To whom does she feel accountable?

Is she willing to take risks to effect change in maternity care? By being a risk taker she helps turn dreams and ideas into reality. This is not easy, but the challenge of improving maternity care is what drives change agents. One consistent thread running through the careers of successful labor assistants is that they were not afraid to take risks. They spoke out. They tackled situations where the prospects for success were uncertain. They demonstrated that they would rather be challenged and take a risk than be safe and bored. They possessed self-confidence. They were able to substantiate why they did something.

Risk can be as small as suggesting an alternative or compromise to an accepted hospital rule. For example, one labor assistant suggested the nursery nurse perform the newborn exam in the room with the parents, rather than in the nursery away from the parents. Or risk can be as large as a face-to-face conflict or confrontation with a caregiver. One labor assistant encountered a potential conflict with physician with whom she'd never worked. She introduced herself to the physician after being hired by a client. The physician made it clear that he would not welcome the labor assistant at this birth. She calmly informed the doctor that if he felt that strongly, he should discuss that with his patient, so his patient would have a choice about keeping the monitrice. Because the labor assistant handled the situation calmly and professionally, the doctor then confessed that he was concerned about the labor assistant's presence at the birth because the patient had several risk factors. Once he had revealed his reservations, the labor assistant told the doctor she had handled many clients with the same risk factors. The labor assistant's willingness to take a risk with this doctor resulted in a birth that was satisfying to the physician, the woman, and the monitrice.

It's important for the labor assistant to determine her goals for working with childbearing families. Developing a goal is the first step in effecting change. With a goal in mind it will be easier to develop a plan. A well thought out plan-- whether it is how to help the baby descend into the pelvis in this labor or how to get the nurses at the hospital to encourage mothers to move freely in labor unencumbered by electronic fetal monitors--eliminates fumbling, dissolves possible roadblocks that can crop up, and helps the labor assistant view the problem in its entirety rather than spotlighting only one facet of the problem.

Negotiation with other Health Care Workers

Negotiating with those in the hospital setting is a large part of the labor assistants role. The labor assistant must create a place for herself in a health care setting where roles have been established for years; this is not easy. It requires infinite patience and the ability to understand the "culture" of the system. Using her power as a positive force to influence others already in that system will help mothers to have the birth experiences they want and need. An association with those in power is also important. If the labor assistant always sees those in power as the "other side," this will hinder her ability to work within the system to effect change. Patient advocates must have a power base in order to meet their client's needs. The labor assistant must learn to work with physicians and nurses, using her power to effect change on behalf of someone, rather than over someone.

Penny Simkin, PT, experienced childbirth educator, labor assistant, and author of *The Birth Partner: Everything You Need to Know to Help a Woman Through Childbirth,* sees the labor assistant's role as that of mediator whose goal is to facilitate solutions when differences in priorities or conflicts exist. She feels women's experiences of birth are more satisfying when they and their caregivers work together in harmony and respect.

"The very nature of the relationship between client and caregiver (or patient and doctor or midwife) carries the potential for conflict. Although they share some priorities--for example, a healthy mother and baby--there are others they do not share. Caregivers are concerned about peer opinions, hospital policies, legal liability, finances, time, sleep, and other personal needs that are of little interest to their clients. They are also influenced by their previous experience--negative or positive--with specific problems. Clients, on the other hand, are concerned that their own personal needs, fears, opinions be respected. They also have financial concerns and (as are their caregivers) they are influenced by their previous experiences--negative and positive--with specific problems. Neither party is wrong, but it is obvious that the potential for conflict wherever there are such underlying differences, especially when either or both parties have strong feelings."

"The labor assistant may find herself in such a situation of conflicting priorities. Each person harbors a personal set of needs, hopes, dreams, fears, failures and faults and negotiating is a type of conflict resolution. The starting point are shared values. The most effective form of advocacy is mediation, helping to find compromises that are acceptable to both parties. Sometimes that means delaying a medical intervention (not refusing it entirely) until the mother has had a chance to try other solutions to a problem. Sometimes it means conveying to the parents a doctor's deep concern about the baby's well-being (and not stubbornness) as the reason for wanting to intervene right away. It always requires a perception by the labor assistant that the differing points of view are legitimate, and usually reconcilable. If she believes that, she behaves in a manner that encourages solutions."

Communication Skills are Critical

Knowing how to communicate with others is as important as knowing what to say. Express feelings in an open, honest and direct way. Be assertive but not aggressive. Aggressive communication is confrontational in tone, controlling, or condescending; it decreases self-esteem, and usually fails to get the desired results.

"My client does not want an episiotomy and she doesn't have to let you do one."

Assertive communication expresses thoughts, feelings, and wants directly, and denotes mutual respect between the communicants.

"Susan feels strongly about avoiding an episiotomy, so could we try these techniques to minimize the need for one?"

Offer to attend a prenatal visit with the client to meet her midwife or physician. This meeting will encourage communication between the client and her primary care-giver, as well as establish the trust of both the labor assistant and her skills. It is equally important for the labor assistant to be able to trust the client, for without an honest relationship, she cannot provide her client with quality care.

Being an assertive, not aggressive, communicator means being direct but not domineering, persistent, but not pushy, outspoken but not overbearing and taking charge but not taking over. The labor assistant must learn to represent her clients' needs and wishes while respecting the feelings of other health care workers.

Some people find it difficult to be assertive with medical professionals, perhaps because they have been socially conditioned to be people-pleasers and peacemakers or because they feel intimidated by these authority figures. The labor assistant's success depends on her ability to interact effectively with other health professionals and to communicate with confidence, authority and conviction. The labor assistant should be more concerned about doing an effective job than about speaking out. When she speaks out, the labor assistant must always keep the needs of her client in the forefront. Everything she does should work toward helping the mother achieve her goals for her birth. The labor assistant is there to help create a climate of cooperation so everyone is working toward the same goal.

If conflicts arise, see them as an opportunity to learn more. Do not be intimidated by conflict. The ability to resolve conflicts is an important part of the relationship between the labor assistant and other health professionals. The first step in resolving a conflict is the willingness to confront the issue. After the conflict has been identified, the next step is to set an appropriate time and place to talk. Try to meet in a neutral setting   at a time convenient to both parties. A breakfast or lunch meeting at a restaurant is often much more appropriate than a meeting in the middle of the day in an office setting.

During this meeting, wise communicators will use "I" messages which express feelings.

"I feel you do not take my suggestions seriously at a birth. I feel hurt by that."

"I feel I am making you uncomfortable or even defensive, when I am trying to help my client with things that are important to her. Then I am in a bind trying to meet her needs without antagonizing you."

Always be sure to state the consequences of the behavior (the feeling) rather than assessing blame in an angry fashion. Wait for the other person to respond even if there is an awkward silence. Listen closely to what the other person says. Try to understand his or her point of view. Be aware of body language and non-verbal behavior. Listen carefully; do not think of responses   while the other person is talking. Try to respond in a nondefensive way. Restate what was heard to clarify the situation.

Ideally, each of the parties in this discussion will present alternative solutions. A mutually agreed upon   solution is reached, restate it. It might also be helpful to follow up the meeting with a written note thanking him or her and informally stating what your commitment to each other regarding the situation has been. It may also help to mention a time to evaluate how the new plan is working.

"Let's meet again after Ms. Jones' birth to talk."

How to Deal With Anger
A professional labor assistant may encounter someone who is acting angrily. The following suggestions might help. Be silent at first; let the other person talk. Then restate what was heard and reflect upon it. Try to translate the angry person's statements into "I" messages. For example, if the person says, "You have no business trying to tell me how to manage this labor," translate that to "I feel you don't respect my management and are questioning not only my authority, but my judgment, and this makes me very angry." The respond the "I" message rather than the angry accusation. Clarify the situation and your intentions. Ask questions   about the situation if necessary to your

understanding. Do set limits for the conversation though. It is   not appropriate for someone to treat a labor assistant in an abusive or rude way. If that occurs, calmly state a willingness to discuss the situation when things are a little less volatile. Gather information about the situation if that is appropriate. Always be precise and accurate when talking to the other person. Apologize if appropriate, but don't if there's nothing to apologize for, don't make an apology. Remain calm and try to develop solutions together to solve the dilemma.

When communicating with someone about a conflict, always remember that a professional labor assistant should be treated with respect, because her role is crucial to the provision of quality maternity care. Look upon the conflict as an opportunity to grow. The effort made to survive a crisis or conflict often requires far greater energy than is required for survival alone; this conflict has the potential to make one a stronger person. This conflict involves risk taking for all involved. Each person fears some potential loss and that is frightening. Decide what is worth taking a risk for and what is not. A good support system will help in this time of crisis. The labor assistant should be rewarded by herself and others for working positively toward a solution. Successful conflict resolution, as opposed to denial and avoidance of conflict, benefits both the labor assistant and those to whom she gives care. Labor assistants do make a difference!

"If you have faith as a mustard seed, you will say to this mountain, move from here to there and it will move and nothing will be impossible for you." Matthew 17:20

6.
Relationship with Hospital or Birth Center Staff

Since ninety-nine percent of all births in the United States take place in a hospital, clinic, or institutional setting the labor assistant must work with more people than the mother's doctor or midwife. She must communicate effectively with numerous nurses and staff members. In many settings there is no conflict and everyone works together. But the labor assistant should be aware there are hospitals where she will encounter resistance to her role.

When attending a birth in the hospital one must always be aware that this is "the house of the doctors and nurses." It is their territory, their turf. The professional labor assistant is often an outsider, someone "allowed" to attend the labor and birth. Because of this, the labor assistant must often take the initiative toward developing a good working relationship with hospital staff. She must work hard at helping the couple get the best of what the institution has to offer, and what they are paying for either directly or indirectly.

"Even with the friendliest and most supportive hospital nurses you are aware that it is their territory and they are allowing your presence."
"To allow is to exercise just as much, if not more power than to forbid."
R.D. Laing

You will probably have to go through a period of proving yourself. Nurses and caregivers who are committed to a positive and fulfilling birth experience for every family want evidence that you will contribute to, rather than detract from, that goal. On the other hand, some people are threatened by your presence perhaps because they are insecure in their own role. If the staff sees the labor assistant as an adversary, or a living reminder that they are inadequate, the environment will not be at all conducive to a calm and peaceful birth.

When it comes to hospital nurses, you may find that at first you are wary of each other. Always introduce yourself. Be pleasant, polite and respectful. Remember that nurses love to teach. Solicit questions. Ask questions. Remind the nurses what your role is with both the birthing couple and the staff. State not only what you are there to do but what you will not do. Try to be as cooperative as possible without undermining your client. If the labor assistant treats the nurses with respect she is much more apt to gain their respect and acceptance. Most labor and delivery nurses meet the mother for the first time during labor and mother and nurse must establish a rapport quickly in an extremely chaotic time. The professional labor assistant helps bridge this gap by knowing both mother and nurse prior to labor. The labor assistant has a prenatal interview with the birthing family to assess their needs and expectations. She already has a relationship with the hospital staff and her presence makes it much easier for the mother and nurse to develop a working relationship quickly. When the doula or monitrice greets the doula by exclaiming, "Hi Ana, I'm glad to see you again" the mother automatically feels safer . When the doula or monitrice is able to present data and information about the laboring couple and their individual situation, it also makes it much easier for the nurse. The professional labor assistant does not in any way replace the nurse or take over nursing tasks; she is there to be with the mother continuously and that in itself helps the nurse. A doula or monitrice is often the only health care provider who is able to provide care for the mother continuously and nurses are often need to care for more than one patient at a time. The nurse has tasks other than supportive care such as charting, medication administration and maternal and fetal assessment. When the nurse is called out of the room to attend to another nursing task she rests easier knowing that the doula's presence and emotional support helps fill the void of her absence.   It's also helpful to reassure the hospital staff by your actions and words that you are not trying to take their jobs away from them. However, there will be times when the best the labor assistant can hope for, is tolerance of her presence.

"They simply tolerate me. I am aware that they talk about me behind my back. They are very quick to criticize me or my actions but will not deal with me openly about it."

"My relationship with hospital staff varies from hostility and scorn to very accepting and grateful for my presence."

When asked how she was able to deal with hospital staff, one successful labor assistant commented that hospital staff did not frighten her. She knew that her responsibility was to her client and if she kept that in mind, she would always do the right thing. Labor assistants need to be confident in their point of view and able to substantiate why they want to do something. They must have the fortitude to be able to recommend what might be unpopular solutions to situations at hand.

One way to open up avenues for a good relationship with hospital staff is to offer to do an inservice program for all the nurses on the role of the professional labor assistant. Prepare a presentation and encourage questions. Labor assistants who have done this generally find the nurses are interested. If you are unable to present an inservice program, you might consider writing a letter to the staff explaining your services. Ask that the letter be presented at a staff meeting and then posted on the nurse's bulletin board.

After a birth where the staff has been helpful write a note to the head nurse or supervisor commenting on the excellence in care. Ask your client to do the same. Do this frequently, when appropriate. Nurses in the labor and delivery setting often don't have any future contact with the mothers they care for and don't have the opportunity for feedback on the care they give.

Some labor assistants find that previous employment at the hospital makes them more acceptable to hospital staff.

"I worked for the hospital before becoming a labor assistant, so I am not looked upon as an outsider."

"My relationship with the hospital staff is an exceptional one and I feel very lucky. I had worked in the hospital for twelve years doing inpatient teaching to high risk clients prior to becoming a monitrice and the nurses were already very comfortable with me."

Sometimes doulas, who simply provide emotional support and are not there in a medical capacity, are less threatening to the nurses.

"The nurses were at first unsure of my role, but when they realized that I was there for the comfort needs of the mom and not medical needs they became very supportive."

Other doulas find the nurses perceive their lack of medical knowledge as a negative.

"The nurses are tolerant of us but talk about us behind our backs. They will not involve us in any decisions despite our efforts to be helpful. They feel that since we are non-nurses we are not qualified to be there."

The doula or monitrice should keep up on the current medical literature by subscribing to medical, nursing and midwifery journals, doula, perinatal nurse and midwifery list serves on the internet. A local group of professional labor assistants could also form a journal club as a way to keep up with her profession. It is important for both doulas and monitrices to keep up with current medical literature. Nothing works more effectively to establish the credibility of the labor assistant than being able to quote from the medical literature.

It is important for the labor assistant to communicate to the staff that she is there to support and assist the laboring couple, not to impose her own values and preferences. Always remember that the birth is the mother's not ours. When nurses and professional labor assistants work together to help the couple their combined efforts are much more effective than either of them working alone. You may find the nurses often welcome an extra hand.

Although sometimes difficult, it is possible to fully represent your client's wishes without alienating the staff. Kind words go a long way. Take time to thank and express appreciation to the staff when they are being   cooperative and helpful. Staff nurses are often underpaid, overworked, and underappreciated. Many nurses are very frustrated about the administrative and paperwork aspects of their job and wish they could spend more time actually caring for the laboring mother. They will be more accepting of you if you see them in a positive light and recognize them as valuable to the mother. When you respect the nurses, they are much more likely to respect and value your presence. Actions like writing a thank you notes when the nurse helpful to you and your client, giving small thank gifts, and gifts of food are nice ways to say "I value your work."

"My relationship with the staff is generally good; they really don't have the inclination to do labor support and so seem to be thankful for my care. I am careful about not getting in their way. Some nurses seem intimidated but I work very hard to keep feelings high."

"I feel the nurses appreciate me and my efforts."

"When my husband was in the same hospital in ICU my relationship with the hospital staff was a life saver to me. The labor and delivery nurses went out of their way to let me sleep for a few hours in a vacant room."

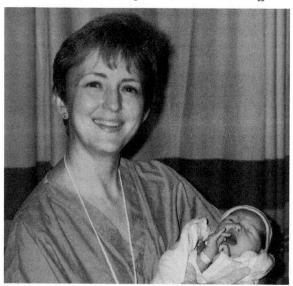

The author, holding her niece,
immediately after assisting at her birth.

Even after much work on your part, you may still find the sentiment about your role is mixed.

"Some nurses are very nice and some are nasty."

"I find that I am either accepted or pushed aside; there's no in-between."

You'll probably find the vast majority of time there is a spirit of teamwork, the rapport is excellent, and only a few nurses   act indifferently.

"The hospital nurses are generally friendly but are intimidated at times. They usually work well with me but at times I notice that they simply stay out of the room until time for the birth."

"My relationship with hospital staff varied. I worked at it and was usually accepted well. Interestingly, I never had any problems except at the large teaching hospitals where the nursing care seemed less reliable anyway."

Working with Physicians

Physicians are the other cornerstone of your practice in a hospital setting. Some physicians are enthusiastic that you are there for their patients. Others are openly hostile to the thought that another independent professional has been hired by the couple; others are simply wary.

"My relationship with physicians varies from suspicious and defensive to friendly, accepting, and grateful for efforts to help the mother."

"There are some doctors who dislike me intensely. If my potential client is attended by one of these doctors, it could create a problem for her so I give her the option of not hiring me, continuing in the situation with this knowledge or changing doctors."

Some physicians do not care whether or not a labor assistant is there. The physicians who seem to have the most problems working with professional labor assistants are those who are the least sensitive, caring or attentive towards their patients. The presence of the labor assistant highlights the fact that this care is lacking.

"They tend to ignore me. If they get irritated by my trying to help the couple, they will usually tell the nurses to get rid of me."

For these reasons, some labor assistants limit their practice by working only with supportive physicians. They find it best to work with a few physicians who value their work.

"Overall, the relationship I have with the physicians on staff is a very positive one. They feel comfortable and not threatened by me, and I feel the same about them. However, I have chosen to limit my practice to the clients of one physician. Our relationship is an excellent one based on friendship and mutual trust. We work very well with one another and give the client the best of both worlds. We complement each other."

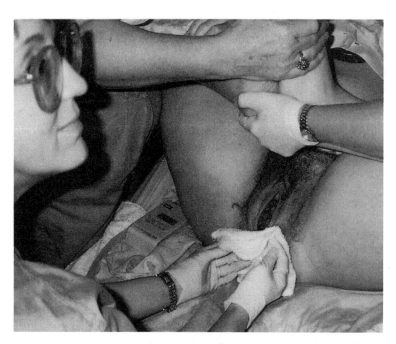

The labor assistant applies warm compresses to help the mother achieve
her goal of birth over an intact perineum.

Some truly supportive physicians have even set up programs so all of
their patients have access to labor support.

*"Dr. Ellis started our program because he firmly believes that every
birth will go more smoothly and be a more positive experience if each
couple has the advantage of continuous emotional and physical care."*

These supportive physicians have found the mother benefits from
labor support. In addition the doctor's and nurse's job is often made
easier. When the couple has hired or invited a professional labor support
person they are much more likely to be well prepared and well informed
and more ready to take responsibility for their actions. Physicians often
rely on the labor assistant for her observations because in many
instances she is the person who knows this couple best.

*"After working with our labor support program for the last two years,
physicians are beginning to recognize our importance in the labor
room. In fact, many have gone as far as insisting that their patients
have someone present for support."*

When Staff are Unfamiliar or Wary of Natural Birth

Even if you have a positive working relationship with the staff, they may not accept the concept of completely natural childbirth. Remember that nationwide sixty to seventy percent of women giving birth in a hospital setting are medicated, and approximately twenty-five percent have a cesarean section. Natural childbirth in a hospital setting is unusual; many nurses and doctors have *never* seen a natural birth and what you are advocating is foreign to them. Persevere and work toward educating the staff. Hospital staff must see over and over again that the woman's body usually "works" when there are no interventions. Your presence in the hospital environment is important to their continuing education, even if they don't realize it at first.

It is important that you have not only a vision but a deep sense of commitment in order to help mothers achieve a natural birth in a hospital setting. Through your compelling vision you will be able to bring others to a place they have not been before. You must be able to teach both parents and professionals why natural birth is best for both mother and baby, when their primary focus is on what is easiest. Natural birth is not easy.

Why choose the hard work and pain of a natural birth rather than the relative ease of a medicated birth? When mother and baby are healthy, and the progress of labor is normal, there are many reasons for a woman to attempt a natural delivery. See the box below for a list of advantages.

Advantages of Natural Birth

- Natural birth is hard, but a woman's body is designed for this function. When a woman births without drugs, anesthesia or medical interventions she learns that she is strong and powerful. She learns self-confidence. She learns to trust herself, even in the face of powerful authority figures.
- Once she realizes her own strength and power, she will have a different attitude, for the rest of her life, about pain, illness, disease, fatigue, and hard or difficult situations.
- When a mother births without drugs, anesthesia, or medical interventions she will approach mothering differently. She will realize that it took hard work to bring this child into the world and it will take hard work to raise this child into an adult.

Advantages of Natural Birth

- Through all of this she will grow as a person, becoming more confident in her abilities to handle any situation that she might face and more responsible for her own destiny.
- Natural birth allows the mother a larger range of options in terms of places to birth, positions for birth, the caregiver attending the birth, and how the delivery is conducted. This allows a woman an internal locus of control (she makes decisions) versus an external locus of control (caregiver or hospital makes decisions).
- Natural birth is medically safer for mother and baby. Anesthesia and other interventions present risks to their health, which include:
  Decrease in maternal blood pressure
  Decrease in fetal heart tones
  Decrease in uterine contractility
  Increase in labor dystocia
  Increase in need for pitocin augmentation
  Increase in maternal temperature
  Decrease in maternal ability to void
  Decrease in maternal pushing ability
  Increase in use of forceps for delivery
  Increase in need for episiotomy and perineal trauma
  Increase in need for cesarean section
  Increase in fetal hypoglycemia
  Increase in maternal/infant separation
  Increase in breastfeeding problems
  Anesthesia headache for mother
  Increase in separation from family unit
  Increase in post-partum back pain for mother
  Nerve palsy or paralysis for mother

If mother and baby are not healthy, or progress of labor is clearly not normal, the use of drugs, anesthesia and other interventions may be justified.

You must prepare the mother for the enormous task ahead of her. You must be able to convince others that this vision that you and the mother share is important and worthwhile.

"At one birth I attended the doctor asked the nurse how many births like this she had seen and the nurse answered, "None."

"I am often told that our local hospital's progressive practices are in part due to my efforts over the last seven years."

Work toward keeping hostile feelings to a bare minimum. If you find a hospital environment frequently hostile, you should inform your potential clients of this. Let them know about your preferences of birth sites and why you have those preferences. Try to optimize the environment for both you and your clients.

"If I'm at my preferred hospital the staff knows me and usually tolerates me well although once in awhile I meet up with a nasty resident. If the primary caregiver is a C.N.M., I have no problems."

Unfortunately, some labor assistants have found themselves in difficult political situations. They have been reported to the hospital hierarchy for discussing with their options other than those recommended by the hospital or staff. One doula reports having to appear before the obstetrical services committee to discuss her involvement with a client. Another labor assistant found her name had been turned in to the Board of Medical Examiners for investigation. A monitrice who is also an RN found that she had been reported to the Board of Nurse Examiners and an investigation ensued. Be aware that situations such as this can occur.

On the other end of the spectrum, some labor assistants have even been able to develop a relationship with the staff so positive, the staff will refer clients to them.

"I have good rapport at my local hospital. Many of the nurses will call me if a mother is having a problem in labor and they are too busy to give her the care that they know she needs."
"The staff tells me that they wish I could be there all the time, but I do have to keep reminding them that I am not there to be a labor and delivery nurse."

If you find after much effort on your part that the staff is still wary of you and your role, simply try to do the best you can, but make sure your clients are aware potential conflicts between you and the staff as well as how you will deal with them. If you find the situation is intolerable you will have to make a decision about whether to continue to attend births at that institution.

"The hospital staff will not support labor assistants unless they know them personally. If they don't let us in, they don't know us. It's a Catch-22."

Enlisting Physicians' and Nurses' Support

Continue to work at empowering both the physician's and nurses' efforts in working with the parents toward the mother's goals. You can do this by focusing your efforts on four themes.

1) *Help the staff to realize how significant they are to the mother.*

As Penny Simkin says, "women never forget their birth experiences, nor the people who care for them. All of us who work with laboring women have a choice in how we will be remembered--as a caring, concerned individual, who said the right things and helped the mother, or the cold, negative one who made it all more difficult than it needed to be." Simkin suggests that caregivers and others ask themselves during the tough times in labor, "how will she remember this?" When one is aware of the permanence of the memory, he or she is more likely to make it a good one.

2) *Make the staff feel special to you.*

Let them you know you are glad they are the ones caring for your client. You can convey that by telling your client in the nurse's presence) something nice about the nurse, if you know anything about her; or you might strike up a conversation with the nurse which communicates your pleasure at working with her: "How long have you worked here?" "I hear the nursing staff is excellent.", or "This hospital has such a good reputation. I am glad we're here with you." Then, as part of your conversation, you might ask the nurse if she has had much experience with natural birth (or VBAC or whatever is your client's choice) and tell her you'd like to work with her on it.

3) *Recognize that all of those involved are part of the same team.*

Help them see that we are all working toward the same goal-safe and fulfilling childbirth. All those working with the mother are part of a team and must feel a part of the team. You do not have to know or like each other to feel this common goal. Help them see that the birth this mother wants is both sane and reasonable and that it takes all of us to help her achieve her goal. Show your appreciation for each person's contribution.

4) *Convey the excitement and rewards of the work.*

As someone who is acting as a leader, you are pulling rather than pushing people toward a goal. You will attract and energize both doctors and nurses to enroll in your exciting vision of childbirth if you are open, accepting, encouraging, cooperative, trusting, and recognize the work of others . Convince them that working with mothers who are desirous of natural birth is infinitely more stimulating, challenging, fascinating and fun than working with mothers who check both their brain and body at the door. Help them to identify with the mother who wants a natural birth. Help them love to work with these mothers and believe in their ability to birth their child.

Birth Centers as the Place for Natural Birth

The best institutional setting for the labor assistant may be the birth center, because the nurses who choose to work in this alternative to hospital birth are likely to be very supportive of natural birth. Monitrices and doulas report their role is more readily accepted there.

"I find the birth center staff to be a striking contrast to the hospital staff."

"When I go to a birth in a hospital setting, I always worry about possible conflicts over what the parents want. It's always so nice to be at the birth center where everyone is on the same wavelength."

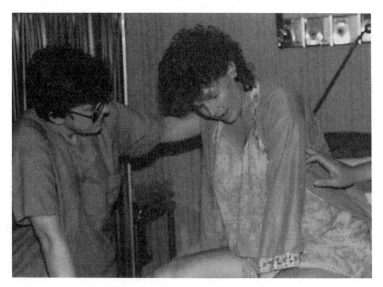

...helping women to discover and draw on their strength.

7.
Psychological Issues of Pregnancy

This following scenario may not be typical, but it does happen and it happens often. A laboring woman and her husband enter the hospital, only to discover their physician will not be there to deliver their child. His partner is on call. Although they had accepted that possibility when they chose their doctor, they didn't think it would happen to them. Their baby will probably be delivered by the partner, a doctor the mother has only met once. The mother and father are cared for by a hospital nurse, who they begin to like, trust, and depend on within a few hours. However, just as the mother seems to be entering a difficult stage of labor, the hospital nurse has to go home for the day. Her shift is over. The next nurse says she can only come in periodically to check on them. It's busy in labor and delivery at this time.

Despite these distractions, the mother delivers her infant son vaginally. She and her husband, marvel at their new baby for a while before he is taken to the newborn nursery for a routine health check. The excitement and drama of the delivery is over, the doctor is gone, the hospital nurse is caring for another couple, and mother and dad are alone.

Although our mom and dad had a normal birth, their son was healthy, and the mother delivered vaginally, their experience illustrates the one aspect of our highly efficient and technical maternity care field that is often neglected. Even in the best of situations, continuity of care is difficult to achieve. But a professional labor assistant can help smooth the ups and downs of our current maternity care system. When a physician other than the mother's primary care-giver delivers the baby, it isn't as unnerving to the parents if a labor assistant, who has grown to know the couple, is there. When hospital nurses change shifts at awkward times for the mother, it isn't as upsetting to the woman if a labor assistant, who knows the mother's needs, is there. When medical interventions seem necessary, it isn't as frightening for the parents, if a labor assistant, who knows the couple's birth plan, can explain the interventions more fully, and can offer alternatives when feasible, is there. The labor assistant is the one person who is there for the parents, before the birth, during the birth and after the birth.

The labor assistant provides, not only continuity of care, but she may be the only person who takes the time to really listen to the mother. She may be the only one adept at dealing with emotional issues which could affect the pregnancy. Some labor assistants see the mother early in pregnancy, some later in the pregnancy, and occasionally only during labor and delivery. Whatever the case, the labor assistant should be prepared to help the mother deal with emotional issues that might make labor more difficult.

Unresolved Issues

When you first meet the mother you will want to learn about possible emotional issues which may affect this pregnancy. When you take the initial history, be sure to ask about previous pregnancies, abortions, stillbirths. How were these resolved? How does she feel about these experiences now? What helped her deal with those experiences? What were her mother's experiences with birth like? Her sister's? It is important to know if these past issues are resolved. If not, they may surface again during this pregnancy or labor.

Mary was referred to a monitrice by her physician during her second pregnancy to maximize her potential for having a vaginal birth. During her first labor she had an extremely long prodromal phase, and a very slow active labor and pushing phase. After pushing for an extended period of time a diagnosis of cephalopelvic disproportion (CPD) was made and her 9lb.4oz. son was delivered by cesarean section. Her husband, mother and father had been with her for this birth. After discussing that birth she was asked how her mother's births had gone. She proceeded to tell of her mother having natural childbirth in a time when most women were heavily medicated for birth. She then went on to explain that her own birth had been very difficult for her mother. The monitrice asked if Mary felt there was any connection between her mother's difficult birth and her own difficult birth. This thought was amazing to Mary. As they went on and discussed the possible relationship, Mary acknowledged that she had indeed had a more difficult process than her mother; she had had a cesarean birth. The monitrice reflected that now that she had had a difficult birth it was possible for her to have an easier experience this time. In fact, it seemed to her that Mary deserved an easier birth this time. They discussed the use of affirmations to help Mary deepen her belief that she deserved an easier birth. She used the affirmations throughout the remainder of her pregnancy. Her labor started with rupture of membranes. Six hours later she birth an 8lb.14oz. son vaginally with no need for an episiotomy.

Eighteen months later Mary birthed again. Her labor was nine hours and it took her only five minutes to push out her 9lb.5oz son--her largest baby to date. When discussing her births now, Mary reveals that as her births got better, her life got better. She explains that she now can be more intimate and she has a much more positive outlook about herself, others and her life.

The Emotional Stages of Pregnancy

Understanding the developmental stages of pregnancy will help the labor assistant assess if the mother is successfully maturing through each stage. Incorporation is the developmental task of the first trimester of pregnancy. The mother must begin to see herself as pregnant. Ambivalent feelings regarding the pregnancy are common and the labor assistant can discuss the mother's feelings with her and reassure her those feelings are normal. A discussion of the importance of good nutrition for both mother and baby is a good way for the labor assistant to validate the invisible body work being done.

As part of incorporation, encourage the mother to become more familiar with her body and its changes. If it's appropriate, the labor assistant can encourage her to begin a physical exercise program. Moderate exercise will help the mother learn how strong her body really is and how she can test what she thinks are its limits. These will be important lessons for her to have learned prior to labor. Exercising may also help her become psychologically comfortable with an open leg position which will be necessary during birth.

During the second trimester of pregnancy, the mother begins to see the fetus as separate from herself. As this process of differentiation occurs, she then begins to attach herself to this newly formed person. Not only is she pregnant but there is a being separate from herself inside of her. She begins to think of herself as a mother and may spend much time talking to her own mother. The ambivalent feelings of the first trimester should be gone now. Uterine dystocia is very common if there are unresolved ambivalent feelings after the fifth month of pregnancy.

Separation is the task of the third trimester. The attachment that began during the second trimester continues and the seventh month often involves a time of preoccupation with the baby. Attachment must take place in order for her to begin now to detach from the baby inside of her. She also should be spending considerable time preparing for the birth. Childbirth education during this time is an integral part of the holistic approach to birth as a psychological development of inner resources. Focusing on the safest way to deliver her infant is important during this time. She must also develop trust in her body's ability to give birth.

Knowing when and to whom to refer a client for more indepth psychological counseling is important. If the mother's major coping mechanism is denial, she may need more assistance in order to accept the reality of her situation. If the mother seems depressed anxious or frightened, if there is much marital discord or severe transgenerational conflicts, a therapist may be necessary. If she remains fixated at a certain developmental stage in the pregnancy and seems unable to progress it may help to have a therapist to help her work through the block.

Dependency on the Labor Assistant

Dependency on the labor assistant is part of the professional relationship. However, it is important that the labor assistant be a facilitator and not a person of power. She should be aware of the "If you're there, everything will be OK" syndrome. The labor assistant must help the mother to develop personal power within herself. The labor assistant should help her prepare to meet the unknown in herself. It is important for the mother to understand that although the doula or monitrice will be there to help, only she can give birth. In many ways, no matter who is there assisting, birth is a solitary affair.

Beliefs, Values, and Their Affect on Labor

Every mother has a set of beliefs about birth. Augmentative beliefs, for example, the beliefs that her body knows how to birth and that labor is good for both her and her baby reflect a very positive belief system. Diminutive beliefs, such as the belief that she cannot birth without anesthesia or that labor and birth will harm her or her baby, are indicative of a negative belief system. In her book *Birthing Normally*, Gayle Peterson discusses in detail the effects of beliefs and attitudes on the labor process. She identifies ways to lay the foundation of self-confidence and mind-body integration. Labor assistants (or childbirth educators to whom they refer the mother) can help the mother attain a more positive attitude toward birth by teaching birth visualizations and sound release (vocalization), using audio tapes to illustrate how the mother may sound in labor and to validate vocalization as an expression of pain. Realistic audio or videotapes of real births let the mother see and hear that birth is painful, and that the pain is tolerable and it is not continuous. They see or hear the woman behaving "normally" between contractions. They also see or hear how quickly the pain stops and how joy and relief take over as soon as the baby is born.

When using audio or videotapes, the labor assistant should be able to help the mother process this information and integrate it in a way that will be helpful to her. Prior to viewing videotapes with her labor assistant, Linda had put aside the thought that she would hurt and had only focused on how beautiful the birth would be. When realistically confronted with the fact considerable pain is part of most natural birth, Linda became frightened. Her fantasy birth had now been replaced with a much more realistic picture. At first this was not to Linda's liking. She was now feeling of insecure and unable to cope. Her labor assistant explained that all women have those fears and that together they would work on ways to cope with the pain. She explained that it was all right to be upset and scared. Linda could use these emotions in a positive way. She noted that Linda had already begun to do that by acknowledging her feelings. Just the act of worrying about how she would cope had great adaptive significance. The labor assistant pointed out that many women are shocked and unprepared for the pain of labor. They do not discover that birth is indeed painful until they are experiencing it; then it is almost impossible for them to cope without the use of drugs. People who have put off the important work of worrying often find themselves suddenly unable to cope when the actual situation occurs. Women who exhibit no anxiety often have complicated births. Now Linda had the chance to work through these feelings and was highly motivated to develop coping techniques for herself prior to the experience. Linda did confront these feelings, learned how to work with the pain, and discovered in labor that she had inner strengths and resources of which she had not been aware.

Linda birthed a healthy little girl after seventeen hours of labor and three and a half hours of pushing. No drugs or anesthesia were necessary. Linda had learned that she could take a difficult task, confront her feelings about it, learn how to deal with it, and accomplish it successfully.

Encouraging the mother to keep a journal of her thoughts and feelings is another way the labor assistant can help the mother to begin to get in touch with herself. A journal is nonjudgemental and is available to her at all times. She may choose to share this with her labor assistant or she may prefer to keep it private and use it simply as a way to validate and record her life experience. Some mothers have used this as a gift for their children later in life--a way to explain to the children how important the experience of giving birth to them was to their mother. Even if the journey through pregnancy and birth has been difficult the mother is able to show her child how much she learned from the experience. Journal keeping may also be a way to facilitate communication with her partner about this amazing life journey. Sharing the thoughts and feelings in her journal may encourage her partner to share some of his feelings too.

Dreams During Pregnancy

Dreams provide the mother with a way for to explore and resolve her feelings and fears at a subconscious level. As part of the initial history or during prenatal visits, the labor assistant may inquire if the mother has had any dreams about the pregnancy, birth or the baby. Mothers often report they dream much more vividly during pregnancy than at any other time in their life. Recall of dreams may also be enhanced by more frequent awakenings.

When asked about dreaming, Robin reported to her monitrice this dream, which she had while still pregnant. She and her husband, Matthew, were standing in a cafeteria line a few days after having the baby. Their friend, Don, was two people ahead of them in the line. Robin noticed a needle hole and brown cleaning solution stain on the back of her own left hand. She asked Matthew to tell her about the delivery because she couldn't remember anything about it. He replied, "That's because you were begging for more drugs." She then asked him why she had been "doped up," as she had very much wanted a drug-free birth. She wanted to know why he had ordered medication. He pointed to the friend ahead of them in the line and responded, "I didn't, Don did." At that point in the dream, R became livid and her voice rose shrilly as she said, "How could you let Don do that? You were supposed to be in charge!" At that point her husband awakened her because she had spoken the last couple of sentences aloud. Matthew was concerned. As long as he had known his wife, he had never seen her this upset.

This dream gave Robin the opportunity to discuss with her monitrice her realization that even though others are there for support, birth is in a sense, a solitary journey. Only the mother can birth the baby. She is in charge. Then they discussed the need for R to take responsibility for the birth and not to turn that responsibility over to anyone else - husband, monitrice, physician, friend.

The labor assistant can also suggest active dreaming to help some mothers. She may suggest thinking about a problem or concern immediately before going to sleep as a way of actively encouraging subconscious activity. Be careful about encouraging this--thinking too much about a problem may cause more sleep disturbances. To help Lea develop confidence in her ability to have a natural birth, her labor assistant suggested that she might let her dreams help her deal with the situation. A few days later Lea called the labor assistant and excitedly relayed the following dream sequence. There had been some kind of natural disaster that produced flooding and she and her sister were stranded on high ground with lots of other people. Helicopters were coming to pick them up and carry them to safety. Hanging from the helicopters were hexagonal-shaped metal carriers that had foot and hand holds built into them. The people would step on these carriers and cling to them while the helicopter lifted them to safety. She and her sister were separated and were rescued by different helicopters. When Lea's helicopter lifted off she realized that she had gotten on the carrier the wrong way and instead of facing it, she had her back to it. This was a much harder way to ride physically as well as emotionally. She was afraid of heights and this position intensified that fear. She realized that in order to get to safety she would have to deal with this fear. She forced herself to look around. She looked down at the ground and at her sister's helicopter. She did indeed reach safety and went immediately to look for her sister. Her sister did not seem to see her as she was running toward her. It occurred to Lea in the dream that this could be because she was really dead and only a spirit. Her sister finally did see her and they went together to see the others on Lea's helicopter. When they got to the helicopter, all the people who had been aboard were dressed in black. They said, "We're going to heaven." She realized that she was dressed in white and that the others had died and she had made it to safety alive. When she awoke she felt a sense of peace and realized that no matter what happened she could birth her baby. She called her monitrice and exclaimed, "I'm no longer afraid of the pain; I can do this!"

Special Concerns for VBAC Mothers

Quite often during labor the monitrice or doula may need to help the mother deal with psychological issues. Those working with clients who are having vaginal birth after a previous cesarean note that it is common for them to experience emotional dystocia at some point during labor. This often occurs at the point where the cesarean was done with the previous pregnancy. Fears and anxieties that the mother may not have been able to confront until this time need to be dealt with. If the labor assistant knows the circumstances of the previous labor, including when and why the cesarean was done, she can anticipate some of the problems the mother may have to face.

Karen had two cesareans, the first during the second stage for failure to progress, the second an elective repeat cesarean. In her third labor, she found herself terribly afraid of pushing after a relatively short first stage. It seemed to Karen that every time her body tried to push it was also trying to pull the baby back up. She verbalized to her monitrice that she wanted her baby to just fall out. The monitrice humorously confirmed the mother's suspicion that this baby was not going to fall out and needed her help to be born. She was very specific in telling Karen what was happening with each push; that the baby was coming down a little, slipping back, and coming down again. The monitrice's encouragement really was a help to Karen during this scary time. Karen remarked that other doctors and nurses had told her with both her first birth and with her second birth, which was a repeat cesarean, that her body couldn't and shouldn't give birth. The monitrice told Karen, "They were wrong. You are doing it. You've come too far to go back now. This baby is coming out of your vagina today!" She then showed Karen a finger measurement of how far the baby had come. Karen then confessed that she was worried because two months previously a friend of hers had had to have a repeat cesarean after a twelve hour second stage. At this point, Karen had been pushing for an hour and worried that she would not be able to go on that long. The monitrice again commented humorously that she, the monitrice, did not have time for her to push for twelve hours or more. She reassured Karen that she could push her baby out in a much shorter time. Karen continued to say with each push, "I can't push this baby out." The monitrice suggested that instead of repeating "I can't" she begin repeating portions of *The Little Engine that Could*, "I think I can, I think can, I thought I could." She also directed Karen to place her fingers in her vagina to touch her baby's head. She encouraged Karen to push the baby closer and closer to her hand. Later Karen commented that actually feeling the velvety, soft, wrinkled scalp of her unborn child and feeling it move as she pushed had been incredibly helpful. She was thankful for the monitrice's intuitiveness about her fear of going on with the birth, the monitrice's persistent efforts to help her find out why she was afraid, and finally, the monitrice's suggestions for touching the baby which allowed her to let her baby come. The monitrice had helped Karen realize her dream of birthing vaginally in an atmosphere of loving support.

Sometimes the emotional block may involve not the birth itself but other issues. It is difficult for many women to deal with medical personnel whom they see as authority figures. Alice's first baby had been born by cesarean section. She had gone to the hospital after spontaneous rupture of her membranes and pitocin was immediately begun. Six hours later she was 1 cm and her physician told her she had failed to progress and recommended a cesarean section. Alice and her husband refused and requested more time to labor. The physician was indignant that they would refuse what he saw as an order and stormed out of the hospital telling the nurse to "document all of this." At no time was there any sign of fetal distress. Instead of encouraging Alice in her efforts to birth her baby, the nurses kept telling her that the doctor knew best. In this hostile atmosphere Alice tried valiantly to labor for three more hours until the physician returned and told her if she did not agree to a cesarean she would be killing her baby. Her 9lb. 14 oz. son was born by cesarean shortly after this episode. When she returned to the same physician for care during her second pregnancy requesting a VBAC he initially agreed. As the pregnancy progressed she found out accidentally that he had already planned to schedule a repeat cesarean. When she confronted him with this knowledge he told her he really didn't want to waste his time with a VBAC and if she wanted one she should find another doctor. She agreed with him and told him she would do exactly that. This was not the response he expected and as she was exiting his office he came out and told her it really didn't matter if she changed doctors; she was never going to birth a baby from "that" pelvis. Alice changed to a much more supportive physician and hired professional labor support. She had learned from her previous labor that the nursing staff seemed to be there more to back up the doctor, than the family. Alice and her husband wanted someone to be on their side if they encountered a difference of opinion with the doctor. All involved thought that was a remote possibility as her current physician was well known for being calm and encouraging even during a long, difficult process. Unfortunately, when it was time for Alice to go to the hospital during labor her physician was not on call. When the on call physician came to the hospital eight hours after Alice's admission she immediately said if Alice did not progress she would recommend an epidural and if that didn't work, a cesarean. Alice immediately became frightened and told her monitrice that she wanted to leave the hospital. The monitrice told her that if that was her decision she would accompany her but that before leaving the hospital, she should try to gain the support of the on-call physician. The monitrice suggested that Alice honestly explain her fear to this physician and deal with the situation in an assertive manner. The monitrice explained that she had confidence that Alice could birth her baby vaginally and that there was plenty of room in her pelvis to do that. A called the physician back into the room to discuss the situation. The physician initially denied her previous statements, but then did listen to Alice and then reassured her that as long as the baby was OK she would not intervene with a cesarean. She left the room and returned briefly only two times prior to the birth. After 7 1/2 more hours of labor and a 1 hour second stage, Alice triumphantly pushed her 9 lb. 6 oz daughter into the world. She felt that taking an assertive position with the physician, whom she saw as an authority figure, was a turning point in her labor. She was thankful she had someone to support her, encourage her, help her deal with a confrontational situation, and most of all tell her that she had plenty of room to birth her baby through "that" pelvis. It was also important to Alice that if she had chosen to leave the hospital, the monitrice would have gone with her.

If a woman is worried about her ability to mother her child, this concern can affect her labor by slowing dilatation and hindering the birth process. Barbara's membranes had ruptured at 37 weeks and although contractions began within 8 hours she progressed very slowly. She was admitted to the hospital for pitocin augmentation. She commented several times during labor that she couldn't believe that she was going to have the baby (her first). Her monitrice began to ask her questions about the baby. What did   she think the baby looked like? Barbara responded that she didn't   know. What sex did she think the baby would be? Again, she didn't   know. The monitrice persisted and asked her to visualize what the   baby would look like. Barbara reluctantly described a picture. The   monitrice asked her to focus on seeing that baby come out of her   body. She told Barbara to focus on the baby, that her baby needed her to help it get born and to visualize that happening. Barbara went on to give birth to a daughter and then confided to the monitrice that she had not really been ready to be a mother and had not thought much about the baby   until the monitrice helped her to focus on it. The monitrice's continual focus on the baby had actually been irritating to Barbara because she really did not want to accept the fact that her baby   was going to be born. The only reason she began trying to describe the baby and visualizing its birth was that she knew the monitrice would not stop asking her about it unless she did! In fact, when the baby was born, her first words were, "I can't believe it."

Sue had two children born by cesarean section and was attempting to birth vaginally when she seemed "stuck" at 8 cm. The monitrice felt there was no indication of disproportion between the baby and Sue's pelvis, and reassured Sue that the baby would fit and would be born. Still no progress was made. She told Sue that it seemed to her that Sue was frightened of something and asked what that could be. Sue looked up tearfully and replied, "I thought I had this all worked out but I'm scared I won't be a good mother." When questioned why that would be so, she referred to the fact that her other two children lived with their father and not with her. The monitrice tried to reassure her that just because her children lived with their father did not make her a bad or inadequate mother. This did not help. The monitrice then decided to go with Sue's resistance and commented, "I think that you will be a good mother to this baby but perhaps you might be right. We'll never know though if you don't allow this baby to be born. Go ahead and birth the baby and if you aren't a good mother we'll be able to tell and we'll help you learn to be a good mother." Sue seemed to relax somewhat and within thirty minutes her bag of waters broke and she was completely dilated shortly thereafter. Without   help in overcoming her block regarding her mothering skills, Sue might have gone on a third cesarean section. It would have been necessary for someone to "take the baby" instead of her allowing the baby to be born.

Care After the Birth

The services of the professional labor support person are not over after the birth. She supports the mother's efforts to breastfeed her baby and to mother the baby. She sometimes has to intercede with hospital staff on behalf of the mother-infant couple.

Molly had birthed her baby in a hospital birthing room. His Apgar scores were 9 at one and five minutes. At one hour of age a blood glucose test was done as part of the routine nursery procedures. Although the infant was clinically normal and exhibited no signs of hypoglycemia, the glucose reading from the portable glucometer was low. The nursery nurse insisted on taking the infant to the nursery for glucose feedings and observation.. The mother refused. This immediately labeled her as a non- compliant patient and the supervisor was called. When Molly asked the supervisor what would happen if she simply continued to breastfeed her infant and kept him with her, she was told the infant could have convulsions and die. Molly pointed out that the infant appeared and acted normal despite the low reading. At this point the monitrice went over the options regarding the infant's care with Molly. Molly could accept what the nurse's plan and send the infant to the nursery; she could discuss the matter directly with her pediatrician; or she could sign the baby out of the hospital against medical advice. The monitrice told M that if she chose the first option, she, the monitrice, would help her get repeat glucose readings done from outside the hospital. The monitrice asked the nursery nurse if she had found any clinical signs of hypoglycemia other than the low reading. The nursery nurse admitted that the baby appeared and acted normal. With the support of her monitrice, the mother chose to remain in the hospital and discuss the situation with a pediatrician. He suggested doing repeat glucose readings in her room. They were normal and Molly and her infant were discharged later that day. Later, Molly's husband admitted that if the monitrice had not been there he would have given in to the demands of the hospital personnel.

Cathy hired a monitrice to help her because of a previous tragedy with her first baby. With her last birth the hospital routine was to take the baby back to the nursery after feedings. Cathy's baby boy was found dead in his crib in the nursery at seventeen hours of age. He had been dead for approximately one hour by the time he was found. Cathy was adamant this time that her infant would not leave her side. She wanted someone she knew and trusted to be there with her and her baby until she left the hospital. Her monitrice attended her in delivery and remained with her and her infant until they left the hospital 12 hours after the birth. Because Cathy knew there was an advocate for her and her baby, she had the peace of mind to rest after the birth.

Riane was glad to have a monitrice who could tell her of her options in infant care. .She also appreciated the fact that the monitrice could do home visits post-partum to assess the well-being of both mother and babe. Riane had delivered her healthy daughter with no medication or intervention two hours after admission to the hospital. She desired early discharge and had arranged it ahead of time with her pediatrician. As luck would have it, her pediatrician was not on call the morning she birthed; the on-call pediatrician firmly stated that all infants should remain hospitalized for three days, and that he would not release the infant prior to that time. In a quick call to the monitrice, Riane learned that should could leave the hospital with the baby but without the pediatrician's discharge order. The monitrice explained the necessary steps in leaving against medical advice (a.m.a.) and offered her support at home. After another unsatisfactory telephone conversation with the pediatrician, Riane and her husband decided that discharge against medical advice was appropriate in their case. They asked the monitrice to visit them at home the following morning to check on both mother and baby. During this home visit the monitrice also helped them obtain the services of a much more flexible pediatrician. Without the monitrice's help, the family would not have known all the options. They might have remained in an unsatisfactory situation, and might have rejected all medical professionals as being unreasonable people.

Listening and talking after the birth is important to give the families feedback on the strengths they had during the birthing experience, and to help the couple process the experience so they can integrate it successfully in their lives. This can be especially important if the outcome of the birth was less than what they had hoped for. Caring for the psychological needs of laboring women is just as important as caring for their physical needs.

Simple statements by the labor assistant during the labor and birth can plant the seeds of accomplishment, capability, and strength in the mother's mind, even though she might not have seen those qualities in herself. This can be done verbally or in a simple note after the birth--a note which can provide ongoing encouragement to the mother because she can read it over and over. While words are important during labor, once spoken, they are gone. One mother who had an epidural even though she had a labor assistant, felt guilty about needing the anesthesia. After the birth, the monitrice sent the following note to the mother. The note helped change the mother's feelings of guilt and inadequacy, to one's of strength and accomplishment.

"I wanted to let you know of some of my reflections on your labor and birth. You had one of the most difficult kinds of labor possible. Many women are simply not able to handle that kind of labor, and therefore, give up on both the process and themselves and are usually delivered by cesarean section. I was so pleased that you never gave up the idea that you could birth your own baby. Your strong-willed daughter has an equally strong-willed mother. Your daughter was not only in a posterior position, but her head was tilted slightly to the side. Your ability to push out a baby in that position was remarkable. You really did adapt to what needed to be done, even when that included anesthesia. Your intelligent decision benefited not only you, but your baby. I am glad that I was able to help you through this process, but in reality, you did all the work. Please be proud of the work you did."

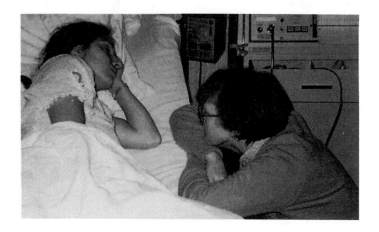

The labor assistant gives the woman
undivided attention throughout every contraction.

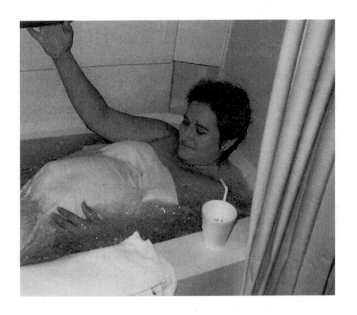

You can even assess fetal well-being while mom is in a warm bath.

8.
Assessing Fetal and Maternal Well-Being

For those who have been working exclusively in the hospital setting there is much to learn about assessing fetal and maternal well-being and providing labor support outside the hospital confines. For those who are new to maternity care, there is simply alot to learn.

Counting Fetal Movements

Labor assistants should teach their clients that counting fetal movement is an excellent way to assess fetal well-being. It is beneficial in all pregnancies, but is especially helpful when the pregnancy extends beyond 40 weeks, or when the woman is at risk with diabetes, high blood pressure, a fetus who may be small for gestational age, or other problems. It is important to convey to the client that observing fetal movements is a reliable way she can tell if her baby is doing well in utero. The technique should be taught in a way that does not increase anxiety in the mother. If it makes her anxious she will not want to do it. Pearson and Weaver noted that only 2.5% of women between 32 and 40 weeks of pregnancy noted less than 10 movements within 12 hours.[1] Therefore, 10 movements in 12 hours is now considered as the lower limit of normal. Any counts lower than this is an indication for more indepth testing of fetal well-being.[2] [3] [4]

Fetal Movement Counting (FMR) is an excellent, easy test of fetal well-being. It is based on the fact that an active baby is a healthy baby. Mothers are one of the best fetal monitors for judging the health of their unborn child. There are many good ways to do it. The method described below is simple and reliable.

Beginning around 32 weeks, a mother should set aside a period of time each day, during which she will time how long it takes for her baby to move 10 times. The first five days or so will give her an idea of the baby's normal range-how long it takes to feel 10 movements. The first five days or so will give her an idea of her baby's normal range--how long it takes for her baby to move 10 times. Encourage the mother to pick a time when her baby is active, usually an hour or so after a meal. After she has established the baby's normal range, she should then be aware if the baby is slowing down, that is, taking longer than his or her range to move 10 times. A mother should notify her caregiver if her baby is slower than normal. (Incidentally, hiccups do not count as movements.) She should count every day if possible, and certainly not miss more than one day at a time. She may use a form like the one below to keep a record.

Fetal Movement Chart

DATE	STARTING TIME	HATCHMARKS	TIME OF TENTH	TOTAL TIME FOR 10

If the baby seems to be slowing down, a nonstress test (NST), which checks the fetal heart response to the baby's activity, or contraction stress test (CST) or fetal biophysical profile may be indicated to assess fetal well-being further.

Some mothers may feel anxious when the are asked to do FMC. They may find themselves preoccupied with all the things that could be wrong with the baby and may worry if the baby happens to be asleep when they begin counting. Try to teach the technique in a way that will not raise anxiety, because she won't do it if it makes her worry. One way to do that is to point out other benefits of FMC. By focusing on her baby for a while each day the mother will enjoy learning the different kinds of movements (kicks, squirms, stretches, etc.) her baby does. She may also learn her baby's sleep-awake patterns and begin to know her baby as an individual. FMC can become an enjoyable part of her daily routine.

When the mother is familiar with her baby's movement pattern, she will be able to use this as a sign of fetal well-being when she is in early labor and has no professional labor attendants with her. When she calls her labor attendant, she can report information about contractions and about fetal well-being. The monitrice should always inquire if the baby is moving as much as it normally does at that time of day. If the mother is unsure, the labor assistant may ask her to count fetal movements for half an hour and call back or she may go to the mother's home to assess fetal well-being.

Assessing Fetal Heart Tones

Assessing and interpreting fetal heart tones is an important task for those labor assistants who are providing more than emotional support during the labor and birth. In the hospital environment, the usual practice is to rely solely on the electronic fetal monitor for assessment of fetal well-being even though medical studies done over the past ten years have shown that routine use of the electronic fetal monitor does *not* result in healthier babies than careful listening and assessment of fetal heart tones by a nurse. Therefore, even those who have previously worked in labor and delivery settings need to learn how to monitor the fetus with a stethoscope or doppler intermittently in labor as well as how to do a nonstress test outside of the hospital setting. Outside of the hospital, the labor assistant will need to learn to use a fetoscope or hand-held Doppler device to assess fetal heart tones. These skills require time and experience, along with a good teacher. Those who are not fully qualified should leave these responsibilities to the caregiver or nurse while they learn. She must be able to hear and distinguish between fetal heart tones, uterine souffle, and funic souffle. The uterine souffle or bruit is the rushing sound of maternal blood going to the placenta and is the same rate as the maternal pulse. The funic souffle is rushing sound of fetal blood in the umbilical cord and is the same rate as the fetal heart rate. Fetal heart tones are distinguished by the presence of valve sounds.

It is quite possible to hear fetal heart rate accelerations and decelerations as well as to determine fetal heart rate variability while monitoring the fetus intermittently. The attendant should count the fetal heart rate for five second intervals every other five seconds and multiply by 12 to get the number of beats per minute. Counts of 8,9,10,11,12,13,14,or 15 correspond to fetal heart rates of 96,108,120,132,144,156,168, and 180 beats per minute.

To establish the baseline heart rate as well as any accelerations or decelerations. This information should be documented in writing. ("baseline heart rate of 132 with variability 11,12,12,11,13,11,12"). One learns to hear what is usually seen on a fetal heart tracing produced with electronic fetal monitoring. Graphing the heart rate is usually not necessary but it may be needed when doing a nonstress test or contraction stress test outside the hospital setting. One might also use a graph simply in order to see what one is hearing. Putting the data in graph form may make it easier for those used to relying on fetal monitor strips for assessment of fetal well-being. This graph may resemble the one used by Paine and her colleagues who assessed the ability to accurately document FHR accelerations by auscultation as well as nonstress tests done by auscultation. [5]

Strip Done By Graphing Auscultated Fetal Heart Rate

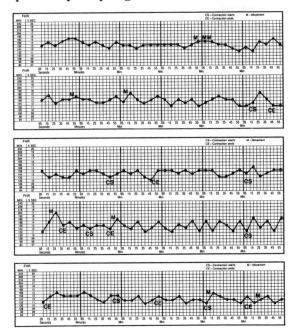

During labor, the fetal heart rate should be evaluated during and immediately after a contraction. In early labor one need only listen to the heart tones once an hour, but in active labor, every 15 minutes. During the second stage, the heart tones should be evaluated every five minutes or after every contraction.

It is also important that the labor assistant understand the physiological mechanisms which control the fetal heart rate, extrinsic factors that impact on the fetal heart rate, the fetus' normal adaptive responses, and variations of the fetal heart rate. This material may be found in nursing or midwifery texts or may be learned from a preceptor. For more detailed study one might consider attending a fetal monitoring seminar, held frequently in many locations around the United States. The labor and delivery units or continuing education department of a hospital may be able to give you information regarding this type of seminar.

Fetal scalp stimulation is also helpful to the labor assistant who is assessing fetal well-being. It is easy to learn and does not require any equipment. This technique is helpful when evaluating heart rate decelerations prior to transport to the hospital or during a birth outside of the hospital setting. During a vaginal examination the labor assistant uses pressure from her fingers to rub or pinch the fetus' scalp, which elicits a response in the fetal heart rate. . Accelerations following scalp stimulation are indicative of a fetal blood pH greater than 7.19. Absence of accelerations does not necessarily mean that fetal acidosis exists but it does mean more detailed assessment of fetal well-being is necessary if delivery is not imminent. [6]

Vaginal Exams

Learning to do vaginal exams for cervical assessment is easiest when working with a preceptor (an experienced labor assistant, a nurse, midwife, or doctor.) Many mothers will allow the apprentice labor assistant to check their cervix each time the preceptor does, then they compare information.

In labor, vaginal exams should be kept to a minimum to decrease the chance of infection, especially once the membranes have ruptured. Remember that vaginal exams may not be comfortable for the mother, vaginal exams ideally just confirm what your other assessments suggest. Each time you do an exam you should have a specific purpose for doing so--they should not be done "by the clock." When doing a vaginal exam, check not only for dilatation, but for cervical position, effacement, application to the fetal head to the cervix, station, and fetal position. Be as gentle and as quick as possible when doing vaginal exams. Always ask the mother's permission to do the exam. Try to do the exam without asking the mother to change positions unless it is impossible for you to make accurate assessments in the position she is in. One will quickly learn to do vaginal exams while the mother is on hands and knees, sitting on the toilet, squatting, or standing.

Assessing Maternal Well-Being

Assessment of maternal well-being is as important as assessment of fetal well-being. Check blood pressure once an hour once labor is well established. The labor assistant should also be able to assess the mother's reflexes. These skills are best learned in an apprenticeship. If one is not sure if the mother has had adequate fluid intake or if she has vomited repeatedly, test her urine for ketones. Readings of 1 plus or above indicate the need for greater fluid intake. Slight elevation of temperature might also indicate dehydration. The mother can drink anything she wants, but keep in mind that citrus fruit juices might be too acidic for some women during labor. Davis suggests the use of a home-made labor drink. This labor-aide is made with 1 quart water, 1/3 cup honey, 1/3 cup lemon juice, 1/2 teaspoon salt, 1/4 teaspoon baking soda, and 2 crushed calcium tablets. [7] Fluids are best if sipped in small, frequent amounts to optimize absorption.

Assessing Contraction Strength

Learn to assess the quality of the contraction by placing your hand lightly on the fundal part of the uterus during a contraction. Contractions are usually rated mild, moderate or firm. The uterus should relax completely between contractions. Be sure you are feeling the uterus and not just a hard fetal part. Share this information with the mother. Be truthful. If they are not firm, do not be afraid to tell her even if she experiences these contractions as painful. Being realistic helps her prepare for the contractions yet to come.

Assessing the Labor Environment

Assessing the labor environment is an important part of assessing maternal well-being. Be conscious of the effect of noise, disturbances and light on the birthing mother. The   birth environment that is unusually noisy or has many distractions can have a negative effect on the birthing mother. It can distract her. Alter the birth environment if possible to make it conducive to relaxation. Some women prefer a softly lit area and others prefer an almost dark atmosphere. The lighting should encourage her to turn inward and focus on the work of birth. If, however, labor is stalled or is proceeding very slowly, a dramatic change of environment could be called for. You might want to open the blinds or curtains and if the weather permits, open the windows. You might suggest that the mother move to another room or go outside for a walk. A change in music (to a more upbeat tempo or to a more soothing calming quality) might help.

Try to be aware of the effect other people can have on the birthing woman. Any negative energy in the room seems to be picked up quickly by the mother. Sometimes it helps to clear the room of all but essential people. This may free the mother of "performance anxiety" or concerns about other people so that she can focus on herself, her baby and her labor.

Conclusion

Many of the methods of assessment described in this chapter require time and skilled teaching before you become proficient and accurate. It is possible to do more harm than good if you rely on such methods before you are fully capable. Be patient and turn to others for these assessments until you can do them reliable. In the meantime, you can still help immeasurably with emotional support and advocacy.

References

[1] Grant, A., et al. Routine formal fetal movement counting and risk of antepartum late death in normally formed singletons. *Lancet* 2(86590:345, 12 Aug. 89.

[2] Pearson, J., Fetal Activity and Fetal Well-being: an Evaluation, *British Medical Journal,* 1:1305-1307, 1976.

[3] E. Sadovsky, Monitoring Fetal Movement: A useful screening test, *Contemporary Obstetrics and Gynecology,* 25(4):123-135, 1985.

[4] Neldham, S. Fetal movements as an indicator of fetal well-being. *Danish Medical Bulletin,* 30(4):274, Jun 83.

[5] Paine, LL, et al. Auscultated Fetal Heart Rate Accelerations, Part I: Accuracy and Documentation, and Part II: An Alternative to the Non-stress Test, *Journal of Nurse-Midwifery,* 31(2):68-77, March/April 1986.

[6] Harvey, Carol J., Fetal Scalp Stimulation: Enhancing the interpretation of fetal monitor tracings, *Perinatal Neonatal Nursing,* 1(1):12-21, 1987.

[7] Elizabeth Davis, *Heart and Hands: A Midwife's Guide to Pregnancy and Birth,* Celestial Arts, Berkeley, California, 1987, p. 71

9.
The Views of Three Obstetricians

What a Difference One Monitrice Can Make
By Douglas A. Thibodeaux, M.D.
Practicing in a small private hospital in Houston, Texas

I started practice in Houston in 1964. I was very excited about medicine and obstetrics in particular, and I was very fortunate to be busy within a short time. Everything seemed fine, except for one problem. I would walk into labor and delivery and hear overly medicated patients who were out of control. I would hear women who had been given scopolamine talking out of their heads. I would put patients to sleep to deliver their babies. Somehow this didn't seem right. I thought there must be a better way. A better way to participate, a better way to enjoy, and a better way to accomplish something that had been done since the human race was created-- help mothers birth babies.

How could I help women have a natural delivery? I became convinced the answer was in educating the mother. But getting started was a real problem. In 1965 very few people shared my conviction that the natural approach was better. I turned to a local childbirth group for help.

I was fortunate to have the group's president enter my practice as a patient and with many interesting discussions, she convinced me Lamaze was the wave of the future. Being convinced was easy: achieving it was a difficult problem.

We had many things to do--convince physicians, convince hospitals, convince patients. We had to change hospital policies to allow husbands in delivery rooms. And then we had to convince husbands they wanted to participate. We had to convince families to be interested in the health care they received. We reached our goal. Most husbands in Houston do go to childbirth classes and they expect to be included in the birth. Many families seek out physicians who are not threatened by free thinking patients. Many patients want to participate in decisions that affect their lives and the lives of their babies. We reached this level because many people put pressure where pressure would produce results. In any struggle, there have to be individuals who sacrifice more than others, who fight longer and harder than others. In Houston, when people speak about individuals who contributed the most towards patient education, Polly Perez, a monitrice, is mentioned as a prime mover.

Polly has helped me in a number of ways to achieve a more fulfilling obstetrical practice. She has taught classes to patients, husbands and siblings. She has counseled my patients and other physicians' patients when they were having difficulty fulfilling wishes and desires. But the most enjoyable relationship I have had with Polly is when she is a monitrice for my patients. As a result, I am now trying to encourage most of my patients to use her monitrice services.

Her services include helping patients establish a plan that will help them accomplish their goals in birth. She gives them practical advice on how to accomplish these. She spends many hours preparing, encouraging and directing them toward their goal of an unmedicated, natural delivery. The goal is usually accomplished, but when alternatives are necessary, she helps the family accept what needs to be done.

Why does this help me? First, let me explain that my goals have always been a successful practice by achieving the following:

- a safe delivery
- a healthy mother and baby
- a satisfied patient
- an educated patient

Doing all of this requires a lot of time and effort, something I don't have in abundance. I realized many years ago that if patients were to be educated, as they needed to be in order to be truly prepared for labor and delivery, I would need someone else to help me achieve these goals. In my case the labor assistant was also an assistant to the obstetrician.

I can't believe that obstetricians are resistant to utilizing the services of very special and talented women like Polly Perez. She makes labor and delivery so easy on me as a physician, you wouldn't believe it. Many years ago when the patient hit the OB unit, she would start asking, "Where's the doctor?" Today, because she's educated, the patient knows she will be cared for according to her plan and my wishes, and when I am needed, I'll be there. A monitrice, by monitoring the patient at home until she needs to come to the hospital, eliminates many useless hours in the hospital. It also eliminates useless procedures that are often costly and even degrading.

Economically, a monitrice's service frees me to do other things. She also attracts to my practice educated, intelligent patients who accept responsibility for their own care. These are the kind of people I want as patients. Most of these patients are successful in their own lives and they bring a certain distinct flavor to my practice.

Recently I set more goals for myself which required utilization of Polly's services to a greater extent. I wanted to lower my c-section rate, to give fewer medications, and to have the patient even more educated than she had previously been. She now consults in my practice one day a week, where her duties include prenatal exams, counseling, and individual education.

Over the years, Polly has laugh me many things. The most important of those lessons is the realization that there are always several ways to achieve the same goal. She has encouraged me to utilize my training to its fullest extent. I know how to do breech deliveries. I know how to do external versions. I know how to vaginally deliver second twins who are transverse or breech. Largely due to her, I routinely attempt external version for breech presentation and am doing vaginal breech deliveries for selected patients. I am doing VBACs and in the last year I have delivered six sets of twins vaginally regardless of the position of the second twin. All of these were achieved with good outcomes for both mother and baby. Polly convinced me it is to the mother's and baby's advantage to do these procedures and when done correctly they carry no more risk than anything else we do.

Many younger obstetricians are no longer trained to do these procedures. In our medical training, our educators tried to convince us that it was easier to do a c-section, but easier on whom? We've also been taught to believe that cesarean birth for breech, repeat cesarean or twins, is less of a malpractice risk for the physician. We often overlook the fact that a cesarean section carries its own risks for mother and baby.

We must not forget that we are here and trained to serve the patient and successfully deliver a healthy baby with the least amount of trauma to both. Polly has given of her talents to help me accomplish these goals;

and by giving of herself and working diligently, has helped many babies come into the world in the safest way possible.

Polly Perez is knowledgeable about obstetrics and she keeps up with the literature. She knows about the newest technology, sometimes even before its available at our hospital. She never loses sight of the primary goal, patient satisfaction and safety.

It has been a privilege to work with her all these years and I am satisfied it has been mutually beneficial, but I have benefited far more than she or even my patients have. I truly feel sorry for physicians who do not or are not using the talents of special women like Polly Perez.

Finding a Silver Cloud that Occasionally Brings Rain
By Bethany M. Hays, M.D., FACOG
Practicing at a high-risk center in Houston, Texas

My first encounter with a monitrice, was to be dragged under duress, into the relationship because one of my patients insisted. The monitrice in question, had tried to care for my patients before, but I had refused on several occasions to work with her. My ego strength, like most physicians', is good (it has to be to get through medical school), but I felt threatened by these possibilities:

- I was not everything my patient needed,
- The monitrice might question my decisions, or worse, know more than I,
- The monitrice might come between me and my patient,
- The added person might make an increasingly difficult job even more difficult.

In short, I thought my patient had probably flipped her lid. Two things convinced me to allow this madness. First, the patient was also a friend of mine from junior high school and medical school. How could I say no to this request just because she was crazy? Second, she refused to budge on the issue and despite my most impassioned arguments about why we did not need this interloper, she just smiled, implying it would really be an act of friendship on my part if I would humor her.

The monitrice, having been drawn into this challenging environment, was, to my mind, doomed to fail.

As we discussed the need for the monitrice, my friend Carol and I went back over her previous birth and our perceptions of what had happened. I remembered that it had been a difficult labor, in which Carol and her husband had used traditional Lamaze techniques, that the baby had been healthy and the delivery vaginal. From an obstetrician's point of view, a total success. She remembered an induction at 42 weeks, exhaustion, fear, a dreadful forceps delivery under pudendal anesthesia, followed by a severe febrile reaction, shaking chills and her baby being taken away for a sepsis workup and intravenous therapy.

Then, days of physical pain from a   fourth degree episiotomy and emotional pain from separation from her baby.

Well, I had forgotten the fourth degree episiotomy, also the fever and chills which, at the time scared me so badly I considered streptococcal puerperal fever and had started IV antibiotics in the delivery room. In fact, having been reminded of this disaster, I could only agree. It had been an awful birth and I was glad I had learned some obstetrics since then. Okay, maybe she did need this monitrice.

I had already learned my first lesson about the role of a monitrice: that she could provide a vehicle for communication between doctor and patient. I had also been reminded of something important which I had known and had forgotten in this case--physicians often view events very differently from those receiving care.

Then Carol told me who else she was bringing to the birth--seven of her of her closest female friends. Well, I later came to view this as a plan which was designed to symbolically protect her from all of those bad events of the previous delivery and I was by then just glad that she hadn't changed doctors to top off this plan and so I didn't say much about this further insanity.

The birth came after some slightly unconventional methods to induce labor at 42 weeks--artificially breaking the bag of waters, walking for four hours, and then strolling to the hospital at 7cms. as the monitrice followed along behind in her car. When I arrived at the birthing room there was utter chaos. I had never seen so many women in a labor room. All busy. Some rubbed Carol's legs and back, some brought fluids for her to drink, one took pictures, one cared for the older child. It was ridiculous and I loved it. Here in this cocoon of living breathing, loving friends, Carol gave birth.

But what about the monitrice and how did she win my confidence?

With one sentence. As Carol pushed her baby out and I tried to support the perineum (and her old episiotomy scar), and the noise level rose from seven excited women's anticipation of the birth, I found that I was unable to get Carol to hear my instructions over the din. The monitrice, seeing my plight, leaned to Carol's ear and said, "Carol, listen to Bethany." Carol's eyes opened, we made contact, and the noise and chaos receded leaving me feeling comfortably in control again. I have since learned that I was not then nor am I frequently now in control of much at normal birth, but I was younger then. Having been trained in the traditional halls of medicine where control is an important issue in subtle and not so subtle ways, I appreciated what was more likely a concession on Carol's part than any real need for me to control the birth process.

It was my first encounter with the concept of a caregiver who is responsible only to the patient, not the hospital, not the doctor, just the patient. It was enlightening and pleasant to find that I could benefit from the presence of this person. This birth was the beginning of one of many paths which I traveled at this stage of my career, all of which have led me to a new understanding of birth, of women's roles in the birth process, and my own view of myself as a female caregiver in a male dominated profession.

The Labor Assistant and the Physician

To gain acceptance by a physician the monitrice will have to find out what pressures affect the physician as he or she deals with patients. The monitrice can then use her skills to reassure both the physician and her client. While it may seem patronizing to say that the monitrice has any obligation to the physician, it is nevertheless true that her practice will be limited if physicians perceive her as a threat or a hindrance. If it becomes a contest of wills between monitrice and physician, the physician has the upper hand. The physician's most effective retaliation is simply to limit the monitrice's access to patients by manipulating hospital policy with regard to labor support, but a more subtle way is to make the monitrice appear a failure in her job using the power the physician has over the patient herself. This can be done by subtle messages to the patient which undermine her confidence in the monitrice, failing to follow the plan worked out between doctor and patient, or undermining the monitrice's efforts by such maneuvers as giving medications or anesthesia when the patient is most vulnerable, or using the male camaraderie with the husband to control "the women." ("You don't want her to risk the health of the baby by going on for hours more, do you, especially when it's just to prove something.")

This of course works both ways. The monitrice can be equally destructive, undermining her client's faith in the doctor and making his or her life miserable. The ideal, of course, is for the monitrice and physician to find a common ground, each respecting the talents of the other as well as the need of the patient to trust and respect both. The physician and monitrice, when working together, are a capable and effective team which can accomplish their shared goals much of the time. When these goals are normal birth, a rewarding experience for the family, a safe environment for the mother and fetus, and the best possible outcome, all parties stand to benefit.

Technology

The monitrice should support the judicious use of technology. At the same time it is clearly the monitrice's role to empower the mother in her job of birthing the baby, since no machine or technology has been invented to do this work as well as she can, most of the time. The monitrice walks a fine line between encouraging her client to reject all use of technology and relying too heavily on it. She gives her client confidence that the appropriate use of technology is a useful safeguard for her and her baby, while maintaining her client's confidence in nature and her own ability. It is useful to me as a physician to have patients who don't carry unreasonable expectations about my ability to avert disaster and prevent bad outcomes. I want them to realize that there isn't "magic in them there machines." In fact, physicians themselves have difficulty keeping a clear perspective on our rapidly growing ability to predict and prevent problems, using the science now available. In our enthusiasm we may oversell the technology to both ourselves and our patients. Sometimes having to answer a few questions which I know have been placed in my patient's mind by the monitrice has caused me to rethink not only individual patient care, but also to revise a number of policies and protocols in order to provide more individualized care.

Pressure from the Medical Community

There is one situation which may turn the monitrice into a liability rather than an asset to the physician. Physicians who work with monitrices often find themselves at odds with their fellow physicians. The physician who uses a monitrice is perceived by her or his colleagues as being too busy, too lazy, or too interested in normal birth. The physician who practices differently is viewed suspiciously by his or her colleagues. In addition, if these colleagues have had unfavorable encounters with monitrices, they may try to restrict the monitrice's access to the hospital. This places the physician in a confrontational situation with his or her colleagues. If the physician who works with a monitrice also makes more money and is more successful, she or he will find her or himself to be the target of further criticism from his or her colleagues.

The medical staff is not the only area from which criticism may arise. The nursing staff may also vent their frustration at the monitrice. The current working environment in a hospital is not always the most cooperative. The nursing staff views itself, I believe, as beleaguered. The nursing profession itself is in transition just as is the profession of medicine, but for the nursing profession this transition is mixed with issues of feminist power in the workplace. Nurses, who are predominately women, are treated as handmaidens and "gofers" because of their gender and for no other reason. Men with the same skills are not relegated to this status. Nurses' resentment of their lack of power may be directed toward the labor assistant, who does not have to follow the same rules.

The malpractice crisis has forced nurses to become the minion of the hospital which provides legal protection for them in return for their loyalty and a large sacrifice of their time. Their time is taken away from nursing and patient care in order to provide "defensibility" to the hospital by precise documentation of everything and by following and protecting hospital policies. Many nurses feel the best shelter from malpractice claims is to simply carry out the orders of the physician and hospital policies. How can they practice nursing, make independent evaluations, make "nursing diagnoses" and institute nursing interventions and while appearing to the legal community to merely be doing whatever the doctor orders? This dichotomy puts them into conflict--within themselves and with the physician and hospital administration. This, and constant understaffing, places the nurse in a position of great stress, little support and still leaves her uncompensated by either money or a share in the glory of healing patients.

Into this environment along with the doctor, (one of the "enemy")comes a new insult, a new threat, the monitrice. Here is a nurse practicing independently, on more equal footing with the doctor, (at least in charge of how much she makes), but most insulting of all, able to practice nursing--real, hands-on nursing. Of course the nurses' view of the monitrice does not include the sacrifices the monitrice makes: time; emotional involvement with the family; concessions to the physician to prevent conflict which might disturb her patient; the threat of malpractice without the comfortable big brother of the hospital to foot the bills and take the risk. All they see is a rival, an enemy. From my position as a physician, one of the most difficult aspects of working with a monitrice is perceived as the one who brings interloper into the hospital to insert herself between the patient and her nurse They don't seem to understand that it is the patient who brings the monitrice. They don't see that the monitrice has earned that position of closeness in a number of ways, not the least of which is not leaving at shift change. Nurses view monitrices as making their job more difficult, a complaint which I have never understood (aren't two people doing the work better than one?), and the hostility causes a major problem for the unsuspecting doctor.

In summary, the relationship between the doctor and monitrice can be satisfying and mutually profitable. Or it can be the opposite--it can be stressful, antagonistic and sometimes even dangerous for the patient, if they work against each other. Clearly, we can learn from each other and by working together, we can make birth the magical and fulfilling event it was meant to be. The road ahead will not be easy. Medicine and nursing are changing, and as in any time of revolution there will be casualties. I pray that neither obstetrics (as practiced in the setting of normal birth) nor the monitrice will be among them.

Realizing a Dream
By Harlan F. Ellis, M.D.
Practicing in a small, private hospital in Visalia, California

The labor doulas who work in my obstetrical practice today are paid professional labor assistants present at every birth. Available to laboring mothers around the clock, they are an integral and essential component of the family-centered care I offer.

I began my practice of obstetrics in the mid 1950's in Los Angeles. During my training, an influential teacher-doctor introduced me to the concept of unmedicated births as the best for both baby and mother. I practiced at a large teaching hospital and county facility which drew patients from a wide range of socio-economic levels. I began training obstetrical nurses who worked in my office across the street from the hospital to act as doulas, or labor assistants, for those patients with whom they had formed a bond. The doulas in my practice continued to be much in demand as assistants, and in spite of friction which developed between them and the hospital OB nurses, the benefits to the patients were apparent.

In 1968, I left Los Angeles to establish a private practice in Visalia, California. I was Chief of Obstetrics at a small private hospital. This change allowed me to develop a family- centered, education-oriented practice in which bonding with the baby and meeting the baby's needs after birth are as important as preparing for the optimal birth experience.

The early doulas in my Visalia practice were dedicated mothers who had so enjoyed their own birthing experiences that they came, on call, as volunteers to help mothers through their labors and births. Patient demand for the support and security of a doula increased. They were elevated to professional standing, began receiving pay and working a regular schedule. This allowed every mother to benefit from their experienced care.

All my patients, and their chosen support person (usually the husband), participate in sixteen weeks of classes, beginning quite early in pregnancy. Relaxation techniques are introduced and practiced from early on, and a variety of parenting issues are covered, including bonding, breastfeeding, safety, health and childproofing information, and other topics. The teachers for this series and the childbirth technique series of classes which follows it are also the labor doulas. This allows for longstanding relationships and good communication to develop during the pregnancy, in many cases. Of my patients, 80 percent birth their babies in unmedicated, prepared natural childbirth. Ten percent require some medication, and an additional ten percent have cesarean births.

I attribute my patients' high "success" rate in achieving their desired unmedicated natural childbirth to two things. The first, of course is the patient and her support person's own commitment, and the second is my approach to the nine month pregnancy. In addition to providing prenatal care for the mother and unborn baby, I view this special time, from conception to birth, and then from birth to the baby's first birthday, as a unique opportunity to educate the mother and father, the new family. There may be no other time in life when individuals are as receptive to information and education. I feel it is my responsibility to make the best use of this unique openness to educate couples about their baby's needs, to prepare them for the birth experience and for the rewards and challenges of parenthood. The messages received by my patients from the obstetrical staff, the nurses, teachers, and doulas is one of caring and concern. The relationships formed during pregnancy form a bond which supports the mother through the labor and birth of her child and continues afterward, with peer counseling in the hospital and "After the Baby Comes" classes at the clinic.

All of our labor doulas and most of our obstetrical nurses began their relationship here with their own pregnancies and birth experiences. The labor doulas are already known to us as nurturing individuals, and their own experience giving birth is usually the motivation that drives them to undergo the rigorous training required to become a professional labor doula in my practice.

We have twelve doulas for vaginal birth support and five doulas for cesarean births on staff at all times. My clinic pays them $12.00 for the first hour they assist, and $6.00 an hour for each successive hour, per birth, as a starting rate. They receive a set daily on-call fee, and are also paid to teach the childbirth and parenting classes. Five doulas for vaginal birth and two cesarean doulas are on call at any given time, 365 days a year.

While the labor doulas know and maintain good relations with the OB nurses, they are a self-contained unit. We have monthly staff meetings during which techniques are reviewed using video and discussion, new ideas and problems are explored, schedules are arranged, and any new candidate is discussed.

An applicant for the position of labor doula is first interviewed by a panel of experienced labor doulas. Her attitudes, her own birth experiences, and her family's needs are discussed. She is acquainted with the demands of the job, the need to be available for night call, to have a babysitter available at all times with practically no notice, and so forth. If the candidate is still interested, and she has satisfied the committee as to her attitudes and nurturing qualities, then she begins training.

The candidate attends and observes fifteen births with several different doulas doing the assisting. After each of them, she and the doula have a discussion about the birth, the choices the doula made and why those choices were appropriate under the circumstances. After the period of observation, she will attend fifteen births as the labor doula, with a more experienced doula watching her. Following each of these births she will have a similar analysis and discussion session.

Once the training is completed, she is offered for approval and discussion at the next staff meeting. If her doula peers recommend her for hire, she comes to me for a final interview. Some of the childbirth educator/doulas are I.C.E.A. (International Childbirth Educators Association) certified childbirth educators; otherwise they have no medical background.

The labor doula is called early in the labor, in some cases as soon as the mother arrives at the hospital. Upon arriving, the doula checks in with the OB nurse and receives a description of the labor's progress to that point. The patient's chart includes an extensive history which the doula reviews before introducing herself to the couple. This history was taken at a "Nurses Interview" early in the pregnancy. During this interview the mother answered probing questions which revealed her attitudes and fears, and family expectations, old wives tales, or anxieties that might affect her during labor and birth. This information prepares the doula to enter the special laboring relationship with the couple with as many clues as possible to the state of mind of the laboring mother. For example, a mother whose own mother, sisters or sisters-in-law had medicated births or cesareans may be fearful and mistrustful of her own ability to birth her baby.

The doula "coaches the coach"--the husband or significant other--as well as helping the laboring mother, by offering specific suggestions on comfort measures, position changes, ambulation, and fluid intake.

My staff and I are committed to the belief that childbirth is a normal, physiological process. Therefore mothers are not prepped or shaved, no enemas are given and there is no routine use of I.V.'s or Heparin locks. I have found that a woman who is unmedicated, relaxed and in control will respond appropriately to offers of fluids by drinking proportionately with her thirst. She will not become more or less saturated with fluids than she needs to be, and dehydration will not be a problem.

Without interfering with the work of the OB nurses, the doula regulates the environment for the laboring mother. The environment should be peaceful and nurturing, but that means different things to different mothers. Some want music, or to converse, or just to listen to the doula and husband talking quietly. Others need silence for complete relaxation. Sensitivity to the needs of the mother is the doula's primary concern.

Mothers in my practice are discouraged from spending their whole labor lying in bed. The doula uses her experience with laboring positions to achieve the maximum comfort for the mother. We encourage ambulation into the second stage of labor and the use of a variety of birth positions which allow the mother to relax and work with the force of gravity to gently birth the baby. The doula's help becomes vital as the baby is about to be born as she assists the mother in controlling her breathing and the impulse to bear down so the baby can be born gently and gradually without lacerating the tissue or requiring an episiotomy.

After the baby is born the doula and the obstetrical staff, including me as the doctor, fade into the background; lights and voices are lowered, and there is minimal interference with the new family as the mother and father focus their newborn baby. Thus the bonding of parents and infant is fostered. The doula remains with the parents to assist with breastfeeding. She offers support, helps the new parents to feel comfortable and confident holding their baby, and encourages them to keep the baby skin to skin and suckling frequently for the first twenty-four hours.

Not every prepared, unmedicated natural childbirth happens easily, and in long labors, or ones with difficult presentations the doula is extremely important. Her specialized knowledge of positions and pressure techniques is especially valuable if the mother is birthing a baby who is in a occiput posterior position. The back pain caused by this position can be excruciating, and even a committed and giving husband may find himself over his head when he tries to help the mother relax and concentrate. It often takes his best efforts as well as the best efforts of the doula to help the mother. They both offer encouragement, provide counter-pressure to her lower back and encourage her relaxation through the late first stage and second stage of her labor.

My twenty-five year experience using labor doulas echoes the results published by Klaus and Kennell (see discussion in Chapter 1). I have seen universal success in improving the experience of the mother during her labor and birth. Labor can be an isolating and lonely experience, even with the baby's father present. The doula is trained to reach out and make genuine contact with the mother. I believe that the continuity of care she provides in the form of a trustworthy, knowledgeable and reassuring presence throughout the labor and birth is of tremendous benefit.

Approximately one in ten births results in a cesarean in my practice. When I am faced with indications making it necessary to perform a cesarean birth, it is vital for the mother and father to have the aid of a doula who is a cesarean mother herself and has experience assisting with cesarean births.

Five cesarean doulas on staff have been selected and trained by other cesarean doulas in much the same manner as the vaginal labor doulas. They teach a special series of classes for cesarean birth parents, so mothers who are expecting to have a scheduled cesarean get to know them well and form a bond before the birth. The cesarean doula provides all the same nurturing as the vaginal labor doula, while concentrating on the special needs of a cesarean birth mother. The doula uses all her experience and skill to ensure that the cesarean birth is a positive and memorable time for the couple. Her total focus on the mother is vital because, with the technical and necessary preparations for an optimally safe environment for the impending surgical birth, the emotional needs of the mother and father might otherwise be overlooked.

The cesarean doula travels with the mother to the surgical suite and remains with her, talking her through the administration of the anesthetic. After the anesthetic is fixed, she leaves the mother for a short period, during which time I make contact with her and explain the procedure, offering what reassurance I can. The cesarean doula also deals with concerned family members who might be waiting during the surgery.

While the surgery is being completed, the father and the doula take the baby to the nursery so the pediatrician can perform a more complete examination. After this, the doula helps the father remove his gown and shirt, and sit in a cozy, overstuffed rocker in the nursery with the baby, holding the baby skin to skin. The father bonds with the baby until the new mother leaves the surgery suite.

As in a vaginal birth, the doula does no more or less than the couple needs her to do. For some, a cesarean is a shock, a let down, an emotional ordeal. If that is the case, she will be there to provide support, encouragement, and an experienced ear. She will also film the father and baby bonding, and go give the happy news to the waiting relatives, bringing them down to watch through the nursery window. Siblings are invited to come in and share in the special bonding time.

It is common for the doula to pay a follow-up visit to the mother the next day. They review the experience, discuss the mother's feelings, and her special needs as she recovers from the surgery and adjusts to being the mother of a newborn with needs that don't wait. Again, her own experience as a cesarean mother gives her a wealth of understanding to share with the new mother.

Fifty to sixty percent of women who would once have had a subsequent scheduled cesarean birth now birth their babies naturally in our Vaginal Birth After Cesarean (VBAC) Program. These mothers and their support persons attend the classes for natural childbirth, learning and practicing all the breathing and relaxation techniques. These patients have reason to have heightened fear and anxiety, and the doula must help them address their concerns and help them focus, one contraction at a time, on birthing the baby. Most of our parent couples come to the VBAC extremely well prepared, and the doula supports them with all her experience and caring.

The doula, whether for a natural, vaginal birth or a cesarean, makes a tremendously positive impression on the patients and their support persons. I have never received a negative comment about the role or performance of a doula; not one patient in more than five thousand births has indicated that she didn't need the doula with her. On the contrary, the comments I receive, even from my most masterful birthing couples, indicate that the comforting presence of the doula was a significant contribution to the quality of the birth experience. Fathers frequently comment on how valuable the doula was as a support person. They appreciate her help in coping with labor.

One mother, a La Leche League leader who birthed her two children in my program says, "I needed my husband there for moral support, but when it came right down to it, I needed to see the doula's face and hear her voice. She was the only one I responded to. We shared a bond. She had been right there on that bed before me and had come through it too. I trusted her, and she never let me down."

A woman physician who was a patient of mine had doubts about the usefulness of labor doulas. During her pregnancy she and her husband, also a physician, dutifully attended classes. After she arrived at the hospital in labor, I called in her doula. It turned out to be a long and difficult "back labor." The mother got through it, and had a healthy baby after an unmedicated birth. She now reports, "I couldn't have done it without the doula."

I couldn't and wouldn't practice obstetrics today without doulas. They give me the confidence of knowing the laboring mother is not frightened or alone, and is always in the capable hands of a professional labor assistant. That quality and continuity of care should not be regarded as a "fringe benefit," "an extra," but as an essential and irreplaceable part of the birthing experience.

And yet, many doctors, even colleagues of mine, are hesitant to acknowledge the value of the doula. For some this is clearly a power issue--they don't want to yield any of that special relationship to anyone, especially a non-medical person. For others it is an economic issue. They believe, as my female doctor-patient did until she experienced a birth with a doula herself, that the function of the doula is an unnecessary and costly duplication of the OB nurse's role. Some OB nurses themselves feel resentment, and the presence of the doulas can create hard feelings and a political football that doctors are reluctant to field. This latter situation has not been a problem in my practice for the last fifteen years. We worked hard to forge bonds between the doulas and OB nurses, helping them see that each is an essential and valued member of the team, as am I. In environments where doctors are dictatorial and accustomed to pulling rank, the nurses whose egos get bruised will tend also to be dictatorial and pull rank on the doulas, or, in some cases, on the patients. The whole concept of family centered maternity care should preclude that from happening. I am the doctor, the nurse is the nurse, the doula is the doula, the husband is the husband, and we are all in this birth together to support the mother and have the healthiest baby in the best possible way for the mother. When that is the focus, the politics tend to take care of themselves.

I believe the real issue with doctors' reluctance to accept doulas is just an old one in new clothing. Doctors don't like to depart from what is traditional and familiar. I believe that with time the practice of using professional labor assistants will be an accepted part of the childbirth scene. The doula offers not only a continuity of care, but a continuity with our human past, a sharing of experience and a bonding among women which they value highly. That special bond has largely been ignored by the American medical establishment in this century.

More than 5,000 of my patients have given birth with the assistance of a doula. I know they are most valuable assistants. The doula is a partner with me, the hospital staff, and the mother and father, in arriving at the safest and best birth for the healthiest baby with the greatest potential that family can have.

I wouldn't be in the practice of obstetrics today without them.

10.

The Other Side of the Coin: Advice on Some Difficult Aspects of Labor Support

Frustrations of a Labor Assistant
Beth Shearer, Chestnut Hill, Massachusetts

What frustrations await you in a labor support practice? For most people, the number one problem is living "on call," never being able to call your time your own. Although most birth assistants limit the number of births they attend per month, the uncertainty is virtually the same no matter what the number. It is difficult to overestimate the stress this can place not only on you, but also on the whole family. You often feel pulled between the needs of clients and those of your family, not to mention your own needs.

Your energy reserves are not infinite. When you are totally exhausted and drained, you simply have less to give. The only way to avoid burn-out and a resentful family is to provide some times off call when they can count on you. You also need to find ways to give back to yourself after giving so much to others.

Working with physicians and hospital staff is another source of frustration. Some feel threatened simply by your presence. Some see you as a constant reminder that parents think the staff will not be supportive. Others fear losing control; they might expect you to encourage parents to refuse their recommendations or interfere in other ways. Others are simply concerned about protecting their "turf." Avoid adversarial relationships at all costs. Open conflicts increase parents' anxiety and diminish your effectiveness in supporting them. An open battlefield is hardly a relaxing place to labor! If you find a particular physician or hospital impossible to work with, you can refuse to work with them again, but try not to sacrifice your current client's birth experience to make your point.

A third frustration is clients who wish to avoid responsibility by having you take care of everything for them. Perhaps parents express a lack of trust in their doctor or hospital, but won't consider changing. They expect you to guard them from unwanted intervention. Perhaps they have strong feelings about certain aspects of birth, but won't take responsibility for negotiating a birth plan with their physician, leaving you to do it in labor. If you sense these attitudes, confront head-on their expectations and the limits of your power and responsibility.

Your role is not to make decisions for clients, nor to interfere with their pre-existing relationship with their primary caregiver. You are there to encourage them to take responsibility, help them follow through with their plans and goals. Parents must be their own advocates, with your support. If you are unable to resolve these issues prenatally, or simply feel uncomfortable with the situation, listen to your instincts and send them on to someone else. Otherwise you are sure to find frustration and disappointment down the road, both on your part and theirs. Expectations to "protect" them from an unsupportive physician or to take care of the birth for them are virtually impossible to meet. Always remember it is their birth, not yours.

To deal with all these frustrations, recognize the limits of your power. You cannot be all things to all people. You are not responsible for everything that happens, nor can you guarantee that every birth will go just the way you or your clients want. Because of your enormous investment of time, energy and emotion in each birth experience, it can be frustrating and painful at times when things don't go well. Like parents, however, you need not be perfect. All you need expect of yourself is the best you can do in a given situation at a given time. That is good enough.

Managing Conflict With Medical Staff
1990, by Henci Goer, Sunnyvale, California

If your clients give birth in hospitals and you do more than fluff pillows and rub backs, sooner or later you will clash with medical staff. The very nature of professional labor support is threatening to conventional doctors and nurses. Brigitte Jordan explains in *Birth in Four Cultures*[1] that a sense of superiority is built into *any* functioning system and, "any tampering with the 'correct' way is likely to be regarded as unethical, exploitative, dangerous, bad medicine, and the like." From the medical staff's point of view you are a loose cannon on the deck because they can not control what you tell your clients. However hard you try, eventually some incident will justify their suspicions of you. It is simply a matter of time.

If you receive or even hear of a complaint, don't ignore it. The best approach is, "What seems to be the problem?" Beware of answering when-did-you-stop-beating-your-wife type questions. If you respond to questions which presume wrongdoing, you are in trouble.

Most likely there has been miscommunication or distortion of the actual events, and it is relatively easy to clear the air. But what if it's an irreconcilable difference? Suppose you are fostering non-compliance in patients (not that it will be expressed that way,) and you are summoned before a committee to explain yourself?

This very thing happened to me. I advised a client who had ruptured membranes at term and no labor that the medical literature said that in the absence of signs of infections, watching and waiting produced equally good outcomes and fewer cesareans than routine induction. 'I further told her that should she decide to refuse induction, it was imperative not to have vaginal exams before active labor was established. As I always do, I told her to discuss it with her doctor emphasizing that if she refused induction, she needed to be monitored for infection. She decided not to tell him, but he found out anyway. (It's a long story.) After putting up some resistance, she agreed to go to the hospital.

When I arrived she had already had one vaginal exam and the nurse was going to do another because she didn't think she had felt a head. I said that since the mother had ruptured membranes and wasn't planning on induction, why not wait and do an ultrasound scan? They would have to do one anyway to confirm the position of the baby.

Things went downhill when the doctor told the mother he was going to do a vaginal exam. She asked him why and whether the exam could cause any problems and asked if they could do an ultrasound scan instead? Instead of answering her questions, he threw a full-blown, screaming and yelling tirade, the gist of which was, "I make all decisions." Contributing to his fury was that he asked me to leave, figuring, I suppose, that he could browbeat her better in the absence of her sole support. Instead of complying, I asked the woman, who was after all, my employer, "Is that what you would like me to do?" She answered, "No!" and I sat tight.

The baby was confirmed by ultrasound to be a shoulder presentation. The mother agreed to a cesarean by this doctor since the only other alternative she was offered was driving to another hospital. The doctor refused to allow me to be present saying, if you can believe it, that the mother was his friend, but I was not.

He wrote a letter of complaint to the chairman of the department, who wrote me, and when I responded with a "let's get together and clear this up" letter, he invited me to a meeting with the Obstetrics Committee of the hospital.

What I did and why may prove valuable to you. The following advice is based on what I learned from this experience.

To begin with, I decided to accept the invitation. If you are a professional, you are accountable for your actions.

Meanwhile, keep your sense of humor. It helps maintain your perspective. It helped me to think that one lowly Lamaze teacher had a hospital obstetrics department stirred up like an ant hill on a rainy day.

I sought advice from two sources: I consulted a lawyer to see what, if anything, the hospital might do to me and what legal redress I had if they attempted to restrain me from practicing my profession. His response amounted to "It depends," but that was enough to prevent the committee from intimidating me. The other source was a good friend, a family physician with maverick ideas, who nonetheless seems to slide through the system without making waves. What he told me was golden.

First of all, if you are going before a group, don't go alone. Pick someone relevant, but non-threatening. *Don't*, as was my initial impulse, bring a lawyer or reporter. I took an ex-coordinator of The Birth Place Childbirth Assistant Certification Program. You might not want this person to say anything during the course of the meeting, but even an observer changes the dynamics of the meeting. As it turned out, my companion made a vital point. About the fourth time they mentioned the dangers of ruptured membranes and my ignorance of the mother's herpes, she said, "It seems to me that this mother didn't know the significance of having herpes and it was the doctor's job to inform her of it."

Along the same lines of avoiding threatening behavior, don't bring along a tape recorder. As soon as possible after the meeting, make a record of as much as you can recall. I sat down the same day with a friend and a tape recorder. Her conversational prompts helped me recall much more than I could have on my own. And, of course, you keep copies of all correspondence.

Another tip my friend gave me was that the committee might leave me hanging. If they do, counter it by asking what will happen next and when you may expect to hear about the outcome. It turned out, I needed to do just that.

So much for the mechanics of the meeting. Regarding the content, don't be blinded by your feelings. Beforehand, consider what is realistically achievable and determine your goals. Mine were to tell my side of the story, establish that I was a thinking, careful practitioner of my profession, and avoid saying anything that would work against those goals.

My physician friend told me three other things which were of enormous help. The first saved me from making a fatal error. I had intended to show them how knowledgeable I was until he told me "Few doctors really believe patients should make the decisions." He was right. One of the two obstetricians on the committee was a classic authoritarian: "If the woman disagrees with me, she must not care what happens to her baby so I must make her do it." The other, as was the pediatrician, was a more sympathetic type: "If the woman disagrees with me, I must not have explained myself clearly so let me try again." However, neither viewpoint allows for the possibility that the woman has a point of view worth considering. There is no such thing as intelligent dissent or compromise.

My friend's observation is the key to why doulas and monitrices are so troublesome to the medical establishment. They may lead the woman to stray from the "true path" which is unquestioning compliance with the doctor's recommendations. Even questions make the typical obstetrician uneasy--"Doesn't she trust me?" It was clear that the committee members saw themselves as the sole dispensers of information. As is the job of a nurse, my job should be limited to explaining and clarifying anything the doctor said that the woman didn't understand. A consumer advocate is an anathema to the conventional doctor. To illustrate this pint, when I asked for suggestions for the future, the committee replied that if a woman refused significant information to her doctor, *I* should tell him. I carefully said I would take that under consideration, but I doubted that my contractual obligations would permit informing a woman's doctor over her protests. To this they responded that I should consider my contract broken if the woman insisted on concealing information!

The second thing my physician friend told me was "Be very respectful of their power." "I'll show you" invites retaliation. It also goes without saying that you should be a living embodiment of their conservative ideals. Wear business clothes, use controlled gestures, speak calmly and clearly, and speak their language. By this I mean refer to the doctor's "patients" not "clients." On the other hand "respectful" differs from "submissive." You need not, for example, let them use your first name. Politely state that under the circumstances you prefer to be called Mrs. (Ms. or Miss) _____.

The third thing he recommended was, "Go in thoroughly prepared with responses that are well thought out and logical so that even if they disagree with you philosophically, they cannot challenge what you have to say. They may not like you, but they cannot dismiss you out of hand."

I spent time thinking about the issues the committee might raise and shaping a response that met my goals. The prudence I exercise when working with my clients paid off because I could defend everything I had said and done. Further, I thought through what I would and wouldn't say and why. This kept me from being caught off guard even when issues were raised that I hadn't considered.

How did this advice work out in practice? I wanted to tell my story, but I knew that wasn't on their agenda so my opening statement was, "Would you prefer to begin by telling me your concerns, or should I describe the events as I saw them?" Sure enough, the second obstetrician, more open-minded than the chairman, said, "why don't you tell us the story from your point of view?" I wanted to present myself in the light most favorable to the mainstream medical mind, so I described myself as a resource, similar to a book. That is, I suggest questions and alternatives for my clients to discuss with their doctor; I facilitate communication between doctor and patient. They may hate the idea of an outside resource, but how could they oppose informed consent?

The meeting ended with an admonition never to let this happen again. Thanks to my physician friend, who explained it would be a face-saving measure, I was prepared to tolerate a scolding. Even so, I could not resist saying mildly that even were my behavior irreproachable, I did not have total control over the situation. Another friend who knows the people involved and the strength of their dislike whistled when I told her the outcome. Her amazement was a gauge of the success of my tactics.

Eventually most doulas and monitrices limit their practices. I hope my cautionary tale convinces you to do it sooner rather than later. Some choose to refuse patients of certain doctors or hospitals. Others choose to work only with a few compatible care providers. I have chosen the former. Hospital births will never be frustration free for me, but at least I try to avoid intolerable situations. Even so whether you limit your clientele or not, you can't afford to be careless.

References

[1] Jordan, Brigitte. *Birth in Four Cultures*. Eden Press, Downsview, Ontario, 1988. (or) University of Toronto Press, Toronto, Ontario.

11.
Birth Stories

"What a timeless experience. We could have been transported to any time or any place and the experience would have been the same. We were all gathered in that small circle of light to witness a miracle."

...through mothers' eyes
Believing in Myself
Grace Couch, Deer Park, Texas

This is a story for my monitrice, without whom it could not have been written. She believed in me and helped me believe in myself. She made my life brighter. I love her and everything she stands for.

It was Friday night, August 1. I awoke having some cramps and when I went to the bathroom, I saw some mucus. I began having light diarrhea and began to feel extremely anxious. I thought, "I want to have this baby!" After four hours, nothing much happened. I got mad and went to bed.

Tuesday, August 12, I went to the doctor in the morning and she told me I was 70% effaced, 1-2 centimeters dilated, and the baby was at a minus-2 station. At home I began having cramps. I called the doctor, who said I might be in early labor and to plan to go back at 4:30pm to be checked.

The cramps turned into contractions and were close together. I wondered if I would have to have needles stuck in me. Yuck! Would I be able to do this with no medication? I told myself, "this is only one day; I can do it," and I tried to remember how badly a c-section can hurt. I was very glad that J.D., our first child, was at our in-laws because I needed to draw into myself.

Later that afternoon, my husband, Rusty, and I went to the hospital. When we got there, my contractions slowed down and weakened. I worried about what would happen if they stopped.

Just as I was changing my clothes, my monitrice arrived. We talked for a little and she made me feel more comfortable. I was still having contractions and I let them out by moaning. She supported my moaning and groaning, telling me it was good. That made me feel even more comfortable. She suggested that I get in the shower, and that felt great! By then, it was 7pm and we started walking. Then it got really rough. I felt like lying down, but my monitrice said the baby needed to come in the pelvis more and that I should keep walking. I felt weird being in the hallway of the hospital, having contractions with all kinds of people going by.

We went back to the room and I wanted Rusty with me constantly.

My monitrice kept assuring me that everything was all right. I couldn't seem to do the Lamaze breathing I had learned with my first pregnancy, so I started moaning deep in my throat and relaxing my body until it felt limp. Sometimes I was seized by the thought that this was it and I was really doing it and I was filled with a sense of wonder and extreme excitement.

The doctor broke my bag of waters. I went into the bathroom and things started to change. I got really scared. The things I had used to cope before did not seem to be working. After three or four contractions the hair raised on the back of my neck and my body was totally tense. *I wanted out of this!* It hit me like a ton of bricks. My mind was saying "I can't do this, this is scary, I can't cope, and help, help, help!" I started crying. My monitrice, my husband, and the hospital nurse were all in the bathroom with me. They talked to me and tried to comfort me, but I just wanted *out* of this. I hadn't really planned on this type of pain; I had gotten used to the earlier type. I was totally thrown off by the change. I began to beg for some drugs. I tried to look as desperate as I could. I realized how an addict must feel.   Rusty left. I felt sorry for him. I threw in the towel; I wanted it to end. I would take a damn c-section, anything. I wanted morphine, anything. My labor assistant was true to her word; she said no drugs and began breathing very close to me. After several minutes of my begging she said that I could have something in thirty minutes. This helped immensely. I knew I could go thirty minutes. Then the next contraction came and I lost it again. I stood up, stark naked, and told everyone I was leaving. In my mind, I somehow thought I would go shopping and leave all this baloney behind. I walked out of the bathroom and toward the door. Another contraction came and my monitrice, bless her heart, stayed right with me. I lay down and began to concentrate on her. I concentrated on her eyes, and breathed with much anger and force. It really helped. I soon got much better at this type of breathing and when thirty minutes was up I was very, very, very glad that my monitrice was there and had not given in to me. I was coping again and felt on top of it. I was proud of my team for supporting me and I also began to realize that the baby must be close to being born. I told myself "This is the roughest part; I can do it."

Soon I got a funny uncontrollable desire to push. I asked how much longer now and the labor assistant said not more than two hours. I was elated!!! Only two hours. I knew then I had it made. I was excited and pushed and pushed and pushed. I was really working hard. I never sweated so much in my life but I didn't care. I wanted it and I wanted to see my little Cody.

I pushed like crazy and the baby really moved. I pushed again and out came the head. I was shocked! Then I was afraid to look. I could hear everyone talking and Rusty said, "Wow, look at that." Everyone said, "Grace, open your eyes, open your eyes." I did, just in time to see him being born. I didn't like it when he left me; I felt like I was losing a large part of me. But then the most wonderful feeling came over me and such a sense of pride. *I did it!!!* I was looking at him and he was close on my breast all warm and waxy. He was just great to look at. He was such a wonder; so important in my life. I had really waited a long time and the moment had clearly been well worth it. He was beautiful with loads of hair. I looked at him in absolute amazement. I loved him.

I felt triumphant. I now knew what it is like, this unexplainable thing called birth. I couldn't get over how great I felt and how painless my body was. I kept thinking about the birth over and over. I was really truly surprised. I thought of how well my monitrice had taken care of me. I felt so close to Rusty and Cody. I knew I would cherish this my whole life.

A Wonderful Homebirth
Heather Mitchell, Cambridge Springs, Pennsylvania

Labor started when my husband and I were trying to do a belly cast. I thought the contractions were because I was staying in one position too long. The contractions were coming every 3-5 minutes but I was trying to not move and ruin the belly cast. When I finally was able to get the cast off, I got in the shower hoping the contractions would stop but they didn't. In fact, they were coming harder and faster. At 9:15pm, I called my midwife, my doula and my mother. My mother was so apprehensive when we told her we were birthing at home. Having her there for the birth was marvelous and, after the birth, I loved hearing her telling others about it.

At 11 p.m. my water broke and I knew that there was no going back-just forward. By 11:30 p.m. all of my birth team were there. My husband and a friend filled the birth pool and when my midwife did a vaginal check the baby was at a O station and I was 7-8 centimeters dilated. My husband and I settled into the pool and I breathed as deeply as I could through the contractions. I was very calm and didn't need any direction or coaching. I decided to get out of the pool to go to the bathroom and as I got out ,the contractions started getting closer and even harder. After the trip to the bathroom I made a choice to lay on my side in bed. WRONG choice!! That hurt so badly. I got out of that position and leaned against the back of the bed with about three pillows. The contractions were starting to get really tough and I felt I was almost to the second stage of labor.

Around 2 am, I started to feel the urge to push but couldn't remember how so I just breathed through the contractions until I remembered what muscles to use. By that time, the uncontrollable urge to push took over and I pushed with all of my might. I had to make sounds in order to push effectively. I felt as if I was getting nowhere for awhile and almost lost control. At one point, I yelled for someone to get in my face to help me focus on pushing. Then my doula and midwife thought that it might be better for me to push in the hands-and-knees position. I hated that and with help from my doula, I rolled to the side of the bed and onto my Mom's lap. She held me and wiped my head and told me, "Mommy's here, it's okay." I lay almost flat with my head and shoulders in her lap and melted into her. My husband was on one side and my doula was on the other as my mother held me. I felt the stinging on my perineum and I slowly pushed my baby out. I tried to touch his head while he was crowning but I couldn't feel it. With the next contraction, his head slid out and with a whoosh the rest of his body came out at 3 am. I picked him up and he was making these wonderful baby noises. We named him Adam Stephen and he weighed 8 pounds and 8 ounces.

A Letter to My Monitrice
Lori Sisto, Bay Village, Ohio
    The following story shows how a monitrice can even support a mother long distance.

Ah, the first day of spring. It feels like the spring in my life is returning. I feel I can now move forward again..

You'll never know how much you helped me navigate through the crisis and this sadness. I felt trapped having only one choice when the baby died. Then when I called you and you offered me another choice, I felt better. Your doctor friend took so much time talking with me on the phone. I could feel her caring even though many miles separated us. In the end her suggestion to look for a physician with experience with high risk pregnancies and affiliated with a teaching hospital helped. Through a nurse friend here I learned of Dr. V and when I called and explained the situation to his nurse she got me in to see him that afternoon.

When I saw him I explained that the baby had died in utero four weeks previously and because I did not go into labor my doctor had attempted to induce labor with prostaglandin two days in a row. It did not work. It had little effect on my cervix but enormous side effects for me. As Dr. V. discussed with me the possible ways to remove the baby, he was mainly concerned with my physical health and emotional well-being. I had a good "gut feeling" about him immediately--just like I had about you. I decided the best thing to do was a dilatation and evacuation (D&E) even though I knew there was some risk of a perforated uterus. I felt confident in his ability and had a great deal of faith that God had already handed me all that He knew I could handle. I was scheduled for surgery the following morning.

When I arrived at the hospital the next morning, I must have had at least a dozen people attending me because it was a teaching hospital. Some had tears in their eyes as they spoke to me and asked me history questions.

They always referred to my baby as "my baby" not the fetus, "it," or any other name. They were comforting and empathetic. During the admission and preparation time I saw Dr. V five times. He asked how I was and if I had any more questions. He explained how he had to dilate my cervix enough for the instruments and how the ultrasound would help guide him. He said it was a difficult procedure, but then he winked and said not to worry as that was his responsibility, not mine. When I awoke Dr. V told me that the procedure was successful. The baby had been floating in meconium and was very macerated. I was glad that you had told me that the baby might come out in pieces with this procedure, because that's what happened.

Thanks to you and Dr. V for telling us about the emotional ups and downs and how Bill and I could work together through this. You helped us understand that grieving was healthy, normal and a *must*. Just as with our other two births when you were helping us, Bill was truly supportive. You would have been proud of him. I felt so close to him as we talked and he held my hand so dearly. It was almost like I was falling in love with my husband all over again.

Thank you for all the time you've taken with me on the telephone. I felt nurtured knowing that you were my monitrice for this birth/death even though we were thousands of miles apart. I still cry from time to time and it especially hurts when I see my friends with their babies. Sometimes the tears get in the way but I know time will help and soon I will feel better.

All I Wanted It To Be

Kathleen Hardy, Lansing, Illinois

On August 12, 1985 at 12:32am I had my first beautiful child, Shannon. The only regret I have about her birth is the fact that I was not able to have her the way I had planned. They took her by c-section and I did not see her until hours later. I still regret missing those first few hours with Shannon even though my husband was able to see her right away.

I had a very hard time dealing with the cesarean. Luckily I ran into a very dear old friend, Linda, who was in a VBAC (vaginal birth after cesarean) support group. The group helped me come to terms with my c-section and helped me educate myself so I could have the next one naturally and vaginally.

This group is where I met Judy Smith, my labor assistant. She had started the group and had attended the births of many of the women in the group. She was the kind of person you wanted at a birth, a quiet woman who knew her stuff.

On April 7, 1987, I went into labor around 7:30pm. The contractions began about ten minutes apart. By 12:30am I thought I had better call the midwife who was going to check my dilatation so I could stay at home as late as possible. My husband and I and my doctor felt this improved my chances for a VBAC. The midwife checked me at 1:30am and said I was dilated to five centimeters. She thought I would not have the baby until later that afternoon. She gave my husband and me suggestions on how we could calm down and relax until it was time to go to the hospital. At 4am I felt I could not deal with the contractions anymore even with my husband's help. He called Judy and my doctor to meet us at the hospital.

When we arrived there, just seeing Judy's excited smile made both Brian and me feel better. Around 6:30am, my waterbag broke and the contractions got much stronger and closer. I don't know what I would have done without Judy or my husband during this time. They both helped me walk from bed to the bathroom, talked to me, and let me squeeze them to death! Judy never took my husband's place in the labor room. She just helped both of us. I think because Judy was a woman and had children of her own I listened to her more. As much as I love Brian, he will never understand having a baby or the pain. Neither does the doctor. This is why I think women should help birthing women. I think the time at the hospital went fast because Judy and Brian were there with me.

Around 8am, I was dilated to nine cm and they took me to the delivery room. This was a very exciting time for both Brian and me because we hadn't been able to be together during my daughter's birth. Judy helped me push, she kept me calm and most importantly she enabled Brian to enjoy his son's birth. I can't describe the joy we felt seeing Patrick being born. Missing that with Shannon took so much from both of us. Patrick was born at 8:40am after only 40 minutes of pushing. After the delivery Judy helped me breastfeed, since I hadn't been able to nurse Shannon.

Having Judy and Brian there made the birth experience all I wanted it to be. I think I like myself more. I know we could not have done it without Judy. She helped us to keep up our confidence. She helped us avoid procedures that were not needed.

Having labor support at a birth is a must! Brian and I both agree that if we had had someone with us at Shannon's birth, she might have helped us take the extra time we needed and we might have had Shannon vaginally. I don't think the 5 oz. weight difference between Shannon who was ten pounds and Patrick who was 9lbs. 11 oz. made that much difference.

What Makes a Difference
Juliet Brown, Northridge, California

My first child was born by emergency c-section after fourteen hours of labor. Blaze weighed 9 lb. 12 oz. My midwife said she was presenting with her face tilted back, rather than tucked down, which meant that the widest diameter of her head was presenting. I pushed for three hours and near the end her heart rate ranged from 70 to 200. I felt no guilt about the c- section. I really believe it was necessary to get her out. I did have some sense of failure about not doing it myself because I very much wanted a natural birth. Right after Blaze was born, my doctor said that my next baby would probably be bigger and that I would need another c-section.

I became pregnant again when Blaze was 15 months old. At first I didn't really consider delivering vaginally. Ruth Ancheta, a close friend with whom I walked every day for exercise, encouraged me to think about a VBAC. She is a Bradley teacher and has written *The VBAC Sourcebook*. I began reading. Three books that really made an impression on me were *Silent Knife* (by Nancy W. Cohen and Lois

Estner), *Transformation Through Birth* (by Claudia Panathos), AND *Birthing Normally* (by Gayle Peterson). They helped me to realize that I could birth vaginally. I also wanted a VBAC because I couldn't imagine recovering from a c-section while caring for a newborn and a 15 month old. I had to have baby naturally! I began trying to visualize the baby's birth being a smooth one especially at the point where I got stuck before. I decided to welcome the pain of childbirth as evidence that my body was doing something right; that it was doing exactly what it was supposed to do. I decided to welcome each contraction as a pull of muscles that was bringing my baby closer to me, the natural way. I began to feel confident that my body could and would do it.

Ruth and I talked all the time about *why* my VBAC was going to succeed. Her encouragement was very instrumental in my success. Besides my husband, I had decided to have Ruth present during my birth. My baby was two weeks overdue and my doctor wanted to pop my sac to get labor going. I really felt the baby was ready to come out so I said yes to it. We all went to the hospital at 7am on Monday, February 9, 1987. The contractions began as soon as the bag was broken at 8am. They were strong and regular and I walked for the first two hours of the labor. Around 10am it became very intense and from that time on, I spent the majority of my time on my hands and knees, pelvic rocking. I had to work very hard but at 2pm my 9 lb. 6 oz. girl was born, *vaginally.* We named her Cheyne. Maybe the fact that she was a few ounces smaller than Blaze made her fit through easier. I don't really think so. I know that it was my attitude that made the difference. I knew it was going to hurt but I didn't wish for the pain to go away. I welcomed it and let it come. Ruth helped me to trust that my body do its job.

My Support, My Friend
Lynn Badger, Dinuba, California

My labor began about 8pm. The pains were not too noticeable at first but gradually built up. What I couldn't figure out was why my pains seemed to be all in my back. That wasn't how it was supposed to be, was it? It wasn't ever that way on television. The women always grabbed their abdomen and a few minutes later had a baby.

Even though I had gone to classes, this was my first time and I must admit I was sort of scared. I remember they'd told us to walk to ease the contractions, so I paced the house.

About 11:30pm, my contractions had established themselves at eight minutes apart, so, as I had been told to do, I called my doctor. I was told to go to the hospital and he would meet me there. My husband, Dan, and I arrived at the hospital by 12:15am. The doctor checked me and found I was only one centimeter dilated. Since I'd had kidney problems and gestational diabetes he decided that I should stay the night. In the morning he would break my water. I sent Dan home to sleep and settled in to rest myself. The doctor had given me something to ease the contractions and let me sleep, but sleep eluded me. I would rest for awhile and then walk for awhile. I also took a shower. Nothing seemed to ease the back pain.

By 9am, the contractions were still steady but I was only one and a half cm dilated. The doctor ruptured my membranes and said he would check back later. Dan stayed with me all day helping me to breathe as well as massaging my back. Mostly I walked but occasionally I would lie down. Around 7pm, my contractions really picked up and I moved into active labor. I'd thought it was rough before but now--whew! My labor assistant was called and when she came, what a difference she made. Even though Sandy was a small woman she knew just how to push on my back to give me some relief. At this point my husband was glad for some relief too. Sandy was with us constantly from that point on. She gave me confidence and always let me know I was doing a good job. I never once felt like I had messed up in any way. Both she and Dan kept me going--never allowing me to give up even though it had been twenty-four hours since all this began. I was now in transition and barely focusing on anything. Sandy and Dan took turns breathing with me and rubbing my back. The doctor had come and told me that I had a very large baby (about nine pounds) which was in a posterior position. He did not feel the baby would have enough room to turn, but he thought I could deliver it in the posterior position without any problems.

By midnight I was completely dilated. After trying several positions for pushing, I settled in on my side curled up, still needing back pressure with each push. I was in such pain and so tired that I wasn't sure I could push any longer. When I finally looked at the clock I realized I had been pushing four and a half hours. Now it seemed that my contractions were spacing out. The doctor came in again with another doctor and they conferred and then presented me with my options. They could start Pitocin to increase the frequency and quality of my contractions which might or might not help the situation, or they could do a cesarean. They left the room to give us time to discuss the situation in private. I turned to Dan and just plain told him that the thought of pushing any longer was impossible to even consider. I felt that I had done everything I possibly could and just had no energy left.

Dan agreed with my decision and so did Sandy. She never made me feel as if I had failed at anything. Having a vaginal delivery was very important to me but I just felt I couldn't do any more.

My daughter weighed ten pounds and had a cleft lip and palate and positionally crooked feet. Within hours she was taken to another hospital to fix her feet and to find the best way to feed her. I had to be without her for five days. Through all of this, Sandy came every day. It just so happened that her mother worked at the hospital nursery where they had taken my baby and she would bring me reports and updates on my daughter's condition. Sandy also arranged to borrow a Polaroid camera and took pictures of Laurie so I could at least look at her even if I couldn't hold her.

Sandy quickly became my friend and now years later, we are still friends. She was with me during the cesarean birth of my second daughter. She cried with joy along with us when our baby's facial features were perfect. I named my second daughter Sandy and I don't think I have to tell you why.

A birth without a labor assistant is almost like a birth that is all transition contractions. I for one, am glad that a labor assistant was available to me. Since then I have also chosen to be a labor assistant and I love every minute of it. When you see each baby born, it brings tears to your eyes no matter how often you do it.

Caring and Sharing
Denise Driscoll, East Windsor, New Jersey

My first daughter was born by cesarean section. Her birth was disastrous. My husband and I felt very victimized by the medical community and I grieved for the lost experience of birthing my baby. I got in touch with Cesarean Prevention Movement before we conceived our second child and attended a series of classes to help me deal with my cesarean birth and to prepare for another birth.

I was attending a Michel Odent film when I first met Sherri. During this conversation she immediately conveyed her warmth, compassion, and knowledge. She had had two cesarean sections followed by a home birth, and I sensed she understood the pain I had experienced and the deep need I had for a normal, active birth.

Once I knew I was pregnant I asked Sherri to be our labor assistant. Throughout the first eight months of the pregnancy we talked periodically on the phone. Toward the end, Sherri came to dinner and we spoke more frequently. This made us feel more at ease with one another. I was about seven days overdue and each day Sherri kept in touch, reassuring me that this was perfectly normal. When labor started, I found that I tended to communicate the physical side of my labor to my doctor and the emotional aspects of labor to Sherri.

After several false starts of labor, I went to see my doctor, who was concerned that I would become exhausted. That evening, I was admitted to the hospital and given a shot of morphine to induce sleep. I continued to labor throughout the night. The next morning, Sherri came to the hospital around 9am. By this time my doctor was leaning toward rupturing my membranes. Sherri suggested we all go home and labor there. It was difficult having Sherri contradict the physician but basically she was suggesting another alternative and asking my husband and me to make a decision. She knew that we wanted an active birth, not a birth imposed on us. While the three of us were discussing this, I had a strong contraction and my water broke on its own. We all shared in the excitement and the happy resolution to the dilemma.

We left the hospital to find a diner and eat breakfast. It felt wonderful to be out of the hospital, eating and enjoying the company of Sherri and my husband. I even enjoyed the contractions coming every three to five minutes. After awhile, Sherri suggested that we walk back to the hospital. Labor at this point was fun. As the contractions intensified, Sherri was invaluable in using techniques to ease the pain. She seemed to know what would work at any given point. She really hung in there with me. I never felt her attention wander. She also gave Phillip and me time together throughout the labor. She encouraged me to eat and drink, change positions when necessary, and kept telling me that things were going well. When labor became excruciating, eye contact with Sherri helped tremendously. I knew that she knew exactly how I was feeling. As I was standing and pushing the baby out, Sherri was taking wonderful pictures.

After the baby was born, one of the nurses came in and said she wanted to take the baby to the nursery. I had discussed with Sherri prior to the birth that we did not want the baby to leave us. I was in no condition to argue, so Sherri acted as our advocate and told the nurse that we would like all tests done in our presence. Sherri stayed with us for about an hour after Emily's birth.

Throughout the birth Sherri had given me physical and emotional support. By freeing my husband from the role of coach, he and I were able to lovingly labor together. I didn't rely on him to somehow "save me" so there was no tension between us during the labor. I hear of so many couples getting terribly angry with one another due to fear, isolation and ignorance. Sherri's support broke down fears and made me feel connected to her. Her knowledge gave us security.

After we returned home and a couple of weeks had passed, Sherri came to visit. It was wonderful seeing her again. We had been through the most intense moments of my life and she had played an incredibly important part in it. Although she has since moved far away and I will probably never see her again, I will always feel a love for her. I believe no woman should labor without the help of such a special woman.

Labor Support for my Home Birth
Eileen Thibodeaux, Houston, Texas

The decision to hire labor support and who that person would be were made before we decided to get pregnant. After deciding to have a home birth we began to question the need for a professional labor assistant. Then we heard a lecture on the value of labor support. We needed someone other than our midwife who could provide tender, nurturing care.

The labor assistant I chose was also a friend which made our professional relationship easier to establish. Periodically during my pregnancy she listened to my baby, measured my abdomen, took my blood pressure, and most importantly, listened a lot. Often during our discussions she would encourage me to tell my midwife things I hadn't considered important enough to mention.

On the eleventh day past my due date, only hours after accepting that long pregnancies are my lot in life, I awoke at 3am for what I thought would be just another early morning trip to the bathroom. But after two trips in 10-15 minutes, I could sense that something else was going on. By 3:30 I began to have contractions. At first I was afraid to tell anyone for fear it would stop. At 5 am I finally woke my husband. At 6am I wanted someone to be with us soon, so I called Sherri, our monitrice. She told me that she would be there as soon as she made arrangements for the care of her three children.

At about 8:15am I talked to my midwife and she asked me if there was anything I was afraid of. My immediate thought was "pushing," but I lied and said, "No, nothing." Very shortly thereafter Sherri arrived. She brought food, a fetoscope to listen to the baby's heart rate, a blood pressure cuff, and a loving heart. She helped me in and out of the tub, massaged my back during contractions and helped my husband to help me. She also kept in contact with Pat, our midwife, via telephone. I was

241935

CEF

CUSTOMER'S ORDER NO.				DATE 3/6/03		
NAME Hillary						
ADDRESS						
CITY, STATE, ZIP						
SOLD BY	CASH	C.O.D.	CHARGE	ON ACCT.	MDSE RETD.	PAID OUT

	QUAN.	DESCRIPTION	AMOUNT	
1	1	SWB	13	75
2				
3		CASH		
4				
5				
6				
7				
8				
9				
10				
11				
12				

RECEIVED BY

KEEP THIS SLIP FOR REFERENCE
3705

glad my husband didn't have to do that--he could just concentrate on helping me.

About noon I agreed to have my first vaginal exam. Sherri checked me and I was delighted to find that I was 6 cm dilated--further than I had ever gotten in my first labor before I had a cesarean. Sherri continued to listen periodically to the baby's heart rate and reassured both my husband and me that the baby was doing well.

I remember being tired and hurting a lot and thinking about pushing the baby out. I wanted labor to be over, yet I was afraid that pushing would hurt more than labor. I wanted to ask how much longer this would go on, but I knew no one could tell me so I didn't ask. When Sherri helped me into the shower again I stared at the tiles and thought a lot about having drugs to "take the edge off." But then I knew that since I was at home no drugs were available and, besides that, drugs had been the first thing on my trip down the road to a cesarean with my first birth. I convinced myself that it would be OK to keep going but I still kept saying that this hurt too much. Sherri was always right there telling me how well I was doing.

My midwife had arrived and the room was full of people supporting me. I really needed that. By 5:45 p.m. I was completely dilated and Pat told me that I needed to begin to push because the baby's heart rate was a concern. Now, here it was, the only thing feared--pushing. Sherri helped me try different positions but the baby's heart rate did the best in a semi-reclining position in bed, leaning to the right. On my back was the one position I never thought I would use, but I knew when both my midwife and Sherri told me this was best that I needed to do it. After much concern over the baby's fluctuating heart rate, our emergency backup system was put into action. The ambulance had been called and both Pat and Sherri kept urging me to push the baby out. They told me that if I had not pushed the baby out by the time the ambulance arrived, I would be transported to the hospital. Then Pat said she would need to cut an episiotomy if the baby wasn't out soon. That did it! The thought of an episiotomy scared me more than a trip to the hospital in an ambulance so I *really* pushed. Stephen Neil, all 8 lb. 6oz. of him, was born at 7:30pm, and despite our worries about his heart tones, his Apgars were 8 and 9. After I had delivered the placenta and while the midwife was examining the baby, Sherri got an herbal bath ready for both the baby and me.

My labor and birth was painful but it was made more bearable by the presence of persons I knew, loved and trusted--my husband, my midwife and my labor assistant.

...through the eyes of labor assistants

Making a Difference
Lisa Spracklin, Timmins, Ontario, Canada

I received call from a woman about a Birth Plan Workshop I was offering as a community service . As I chatted with her, I explained about the workshop and my role as a doula. She was intrigued about the service and because she was only 16 years old , I told her that I would not charge her my usual fee. She told me that this was second baby and that her first child didn't survive his first week of life.

We met to talk. Quickly, I found out that she smoked and had a "devil-may-care" attitude. She told me that she slept most of the day and was up most of the night. She usually ate only once or twice a day. I told her how to get vouchers for milk, eggs, orange juice, and prenatal vitamins through a community service program for teenage mothers in need. As a doula, this information worried me. I knew that I had my work cut out for me. I kept meeting with her as I thought the base of her attitude was fear. Her first baby was born as a result of premature labor. When she got to the hospital she was completely dilated with a breech baby whose feet were coming first. No wonder she was scared!

One crisp day in early winter, I got a call from her saying that she was in labor and would call me again when it progressed. Soon she called back telling me that she was going to the hospital. I met her there and the nurse assessed her dilatation at 5 centimeters. In a little bit, the contractions were spacing out and by 2am there were *no* contractions.

I passed a fitful night in a chair and the nurse said "Why don't you go home and get some sleep?" I couldn't. I just couldn't leave her. In the morning, her doctor started a pitocin drip. Quickly, the contractions picked up. At 9:30 am, my client reached over and shut off the IV. I told her that the nurse would not like that and sure enough when the nurse walked in she gave my client a lecture about stopped the drug. My client said that she wanted to do this labor with drugs but the pitocin was restarted.

Ten minutes later she said "Give me drugs!" I knew something was happening for her to ask for drugs so I buzzed for the nurse and asked her to check my client. It was no surprise to me when she announced "She's completely dilated!" All of the sudden, there were three nurses telling my client not to push as they were wheeling her across the hall to the delivery room. It was only a few minutes after getting in the delivery room when her 8 pound 8 ounce baby was born at 10:40 am. She was elated!

I couldn't ever consider being a doula as a job. Supporting women and their partners through the childbearing experience is a passion for me . When I help empower women I feel so rewarded.

Labor Assistant by Phone
Guadalupe Trueba, Mexico City, Mexico

One day, one of my childbirth education students came to class without her husband, telling me that her husband had to leave the city for a few days. She told me that yesterday her doctor told her that the birth wouldn't happen for a week or so. She went on to tell me that she was feeling strange today. I told her to call me anytime since she was anxious about her husband being gone.

At 11pm, I got a frantic call from her. "My contractions have started and they are so strong....my water just broke......I am in so much pain......I have terrible pressure in my pelvis...... I called my husband and he is on the way home.... Lupe, please help me. I didn't think this would happen so fast. OOHHHHH!! Here comes another one and they hurt so much that I can't relax or breathe."

I asked if there was anyone home with her. The answer was "No" so I told her I would stay on the phone with her and help her through the contractions. I told this frantic woman that I wanted to hear her slow breathing. I tried to get her to dress so when her husband got home she could leave for the hospital immediately.

While I was supporting her on the phone, I heard pushing noises. I asked her where she was. The answer was "Sitting on the toilet." I asked her to leave the toilet and get in the knee-chest position. I told her to keep talking to me and I kept slowly breathing with her and asking her to not push.

Next, I asked for her obstetrician's emergency phone number. On another phone, I called him and explained to him that his patient was in labor and was making pushing noises. The doctor didn't believe me. He told me that since it was her first baby she was just making a lot of noise.

A few contractions later, I heard my student say she had just vomited. Again, I called the doctor and asked him to go to the hospital so that he could meet the mother there. He said "OK, I'll be there soon." I didn't want to stop talking with her as she seemed more comfortable when I talked continuously and continued to support her.

Soon her husband arrived. I talked to him and said "Your wife is having the baby very soon...... don't panic if the baby comes out in the car........keep giving her support and telling her she will be fine......if the baby is being born, stop the car and put a sweater around both of them." The baby waited to make his appearance until the couple got to the hospital and was born ten minutes later. The doctor never arrived and the resident caught the baby. Her doctor never came until the next morning. He never believed me when I told him that she was having a precipitous birth.

I talked to the couple in the morning and the mother said that as long as "You were talking to me, I felt safe and strong." I congratulated her for being so wise and tough.

A Stacked Deck
Kathy Bradley, Rockledge, Florida

There are many times in the labor support profession where one is faced with the challenge of being torn between two special events. This is a story of one such situation.

When I was hired by Marge and Jerry, I made sure that they knew that I had a business engagement that fell one week before their due date. I was responsible for the first fund raiser for the Childbirth Enhancement Foundation . I went over my back up plan with them and they were fine with the arrangement.

At 2am on the morning of the fund raiser, I received a call from Marge stating that her water had broken. She was aware of her doctor's protocol in this situation. Here I was totally committed to labor support and caught in the middle of a dilemma. As I hung up the phone, my mind filled with options. My options were to work the birth where I would provide labor support or miss the function where the object was to raise money for labor support. At that point, I prayed.

At 5:15 am, Marge called again telling me that her contractions were 5 minutes apart and lasting 60 seconds. I recommended that she get in the shower and I started the 45 mile drive to her house. When I arrived, Marge decided to go to the hospital before rush hour was in full swing. At the hospital, she was pleased to find that she was 4 centimeters but by 11am there was no change. I reminded her that she was in a new setting and needed to "let go" and give herself permission to get on with the labor. I suggested the shower again and next the rocking chair.

To my relief, at 1:25pm, Marge was 7-8 centimeters with an urge to push. I thought that she would be delivered soon and I would be on the road to my fund raiser. The situation would be win-win for all involved. If it had only been so simple. At 2:15pm, Marge was checked and was told that her cervix was swelling. At that same time, the baby had irregularities on the monitor so an IV was begun and a test was done to check the baby's oxygen level. We all sighed with relief when the test was fine. Pain medication was administered to counteract Marge's heavy urge to push. I was feeling very frustrated for both Marge and myself. My staff encouraged me to focus on my client and they would take care of the fund raiser. I spoke to my back-up person and we decided that she would be master of ceremonies at the event. After I got off the phone, I cried uncontrollably. Soon I felt peaceful and headed back to my client's room.

At 5:30 p.m., Marge was still fighting a strong urge to push so a decision was made to place an epidural.. At 7 p.m., she was still 8 centimeters. Marge and Jerry asked the doctor to wait one more hour but gently told them that with each hour the chances decreased for a vaginal delivery. I found myself frustrated again because we were doing everything- changing positions, using the birth ball, rocking, and relaxing. Why wasn't there any change? Birth is like a deck of cards. You can play different games with them but sometimes the deck is stacked against the kind of outcome you want. Marge and Jerry talked with me and the nurse about their other options but soon we all realized that we had exhausted all of them. I reminded them that the staff had worked beautifully with them. A cesarean was decided on, and in another hour, their 6 lb. 10 oz. baby girl was born. After the surgery, the doctor told us that the baby had a brow presentation and that position was what caused the problems in the labor.

Marge was transferred to the postpartum floor where I asked them how they felt about the cesarean birth. Their answer was "We left no stone unturned and feel OK about the decision to do the cesarean."

I headed home and when I got there I found that the fund raiser was a success. So, in the end, it was a win-win situation for all if us.

A VBAC
Teresa Howard, Atlanta. Georgia

Bailey had been laboring off and on since Friday and when she called me, her voice sounded tired and ready to start giving into her fears. I offered to come over and talk with her and give her a massage. After spending the afternoon with her, I went home at 5pm. In the middle of the night, I got a phone call from her saying that she needed me. I was greeted at the door and was told Bailey was in the tub. I went into the bath room and quickly was able to identify that all of the fears from her previous prodromal labor and cesarean birth were seeping into her mind and overtaking her confidence. The contractions were not the problem and her disbelief in her ability to birth was apparent . My job was to help her "lose her mind" and let her body work.

I had brought her a tightly closed, lavender rose to use in visualizations. I massaged her, talked to her, got her to laugh, and reinforced the idea of "the realm of pain is mainly in the brain." She sat on the birth ball and used it to do pelvic rocking. As she was tired, I suggested that she take a nap. We slept on and off together for almost two hours, waking only for me to press the rice sock on her back while she breathed through contractions.

At this point, Bailey decided to go to the hospital although she wanted to soak in the tub before we left. As I was packing up things for her, I noticed the rose and took it with us.

When we arrived at the hospital, Bailey walked right by the wheel chair sitting in admitting and marched down the hall laughing. I was wondering if she really needed to be there as it seemed to me that there was no way she was in active labor. The midwife arrived and suggested that she should do a exam. As she withdrew her gloved hand, she announced that Bailey was 7-8 centimeters, 100% effaced and the baby was at a 0 station. We cheered and hugged!

Bailey immediately got into the jetted tub. When she remarked that she had a lot of pelvic pressure, the nurse did a exam and found that she was completely dilated. The shift changed and the new nurse entered to room to find Bailey smiling and walking around the room while brushing her hair. She thought she was in the wrong room.

At that point, Bailey didn't have a urge to push so we kept walking around the room. The nurse brought in the squat bar and attached it to the bed as Bailey was grunting though contractions now. The midwife returned and remarked that Bailey's pushing was ineffective. I grabbed a receiving blanket and tied two knots in it so we could use the tug-of-war technique. This helped Bailey to get the feel of pushing but the baby was not moving down. Ten minutes later, the midwife suggested an IV and epidural and perhaps getting the doctor to use the vacuum. The IV was inserted and the nurse asked the midwife if she should compress the IV bag to get the fluid in quicker. The midwife answered "no." At that point, I asked if I could get Bailey in the epidural position before the anesthesiologist got there as I have seen it help downward progress. I sat on the bed with Bailey and prayed in her ear, a prayer for her new daughter and her birth. I also called out to God to help Bailey to use this time to let her body birth the baby. In a few minutes, Bailey yelled out that she felt the baby move down in the pelvis. We then moved her into the toilet to push for a while. When the midwife next checked, the baby was at a +3 station. Whoo hoo!! The epidural request was canceled. I knew the combination of prayer, pep talk and the epidural position had worked wonders. After only a few pushes, her daughter emerged and Bailey cut the cord herself.

A Spiritual, Transcendent Experience
Lisa Klaehn, Brantford, Ontario, Canada

When I know that one of my clients is nearing her due date, I always go to bed wondering if tonight will be the night that the telephone summons me from my customary deep sleep. On this particular evening, I was falling asleep in front of the television and decided to stagger to bed around 10pm. It was a good thing that I did not try to persevere with the meager TV offerings for I was jolted awake at 1:23am by a man saying, "Lisa? Sandra's water just broke."

I usually feel a rush of adrenaline as I am gathering details from the dad, and this time was no exception. I grabbed my clothes and dressed shakily, trying to bring my brain to sufficient consciousness and coherence to dress properly and remember my "birth bag." In this case, I also had a drive of twenty five miles to a home that I had never seen. The dad told me it would be the only one on the road with all its lights on! By the time I reached their home, I had calmed down, was awake, and ready to support the couple in any way that I could.

I found the mom curled in a ball on her hands and knees on their waterbed. With each contraction, she would breathe slowly and rock slightly. Her husband provided pressure on her back where it was sore. She looked up and smiled when the contraction ended, but no more than began to tell me how she was feeling when another contraction came. As I timed them, they were two minutes apart, and it was only ninety minutes after her bag of waters had broken with a splash! This made me a little nervous, as the hospital was a half hour down the road. After a little discussion, she felt that if she was going to go anywhere it should be now, while she still felt like moving. And so thirty minutes after my arrival, we were on our way.

We were taken to the labour/birth room of the small community hospital. The staff welcomed us graciously, and were unobtrusive while carrying out the standard admitting procedures. We became a team, the father and I, doing what could be described as a slow dance around the labouring woman. One of us would rub her back, the other would hold her hand and give her a cool cloth. Both parents looked to me for comfort and reassurance.

She had considerable nausea and I felt helpless to relieve in any way. All I could do was reassure her that it was a good sign that things were progressing. The most comfortable position for her was on hands and knees hugging a pillow, but eventually her feet went to sleep. Then she sat backward on a chair, straddling the back. This was comfortable and it improved her circulation.

Contractions continued every two minutes, with increasing rectal pressure. She developed the characteristic catch in her breath while she was groaning softly through a contraction, and upon examination, was found to be fully dilated. She was jubilant, as this was only five hours after she had felt her first contraction and she had expected something much longer.

The first contractions of the second stage were sufficiently strong to let her know that she wasn't comfortable reclining. She had always been attracted to squatting, so she tried it. It was in this position that her body opened up, the pain diminished and she felt very much in control. She found the best way was to drape herself over her husband on one side and me on the other while she squatted on the bed. This meant that I had to stand on my toes to match her husband's height and keep her shoulders at a uniform level. We found a firm foam wedge for her to rest on between contractions.

The mom's face took on a look of joy and serenity as she worked with each contraction. She was totally absorbed in her sensations, which was fortunate, because the nurses were trying to deal with an unfamiliar position. They raised the bed higher, so that the doctor wouldn't have to bend down so far to catch the baby. This made it worse for me, having to reach even higher to hold the mom.

The head was coming, the doctor was not yet there so the nurses were catching. The doctor entered the room just as the top of the head emerged into the hands of the nurse, and he slipped his gloves on to catch the rest of the baby. The cord was too short to allow the mother to hold her newborn without cutting the cord, so after a couple of contractions, she decided that she could wait no longer and asked that the cord be cut. The father cut the cord, while I took pictures. (I have learned this is also a necessary skill for a doula. One must learn to operate fancy cameras that belong to someone else, at an emotional moment, after little sleep.)

"Our" newborn boy snuggled up to this mother and with a little encouragement, nursed beautifully. The mother had only a small tear, which seemed to occur as the doctor pulled the shoulders out. (At that moment you can coach the mothers about keeping their perineum loose, but doctors seem to resist coaching.)

I stayed with the new family for a couple of hours, taking pictures and going for food for "the team." The mother promptly devoured everything on her plate. The parents wished for their baby to be bathed at their bedside which was a novel idea for the nurse, but she complied. I eventually tore myself away from the family, and after going home found that I was high for the whole day, despite the lack of sleep and the emotional drain from supporting a couple through birth. It really is such a privilege to be included in such an intimate, life-changing event. I develop an emotional bond with those parents at whose births I assist, and they with me. We have all participated in a spiritual, transcendent experience which is truly a miracle.

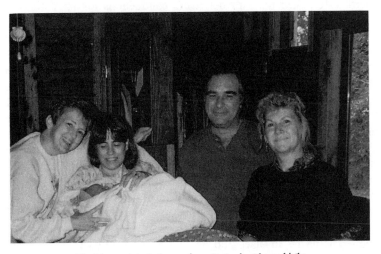

The labor assistant plays an important role at home births.

Primal Instinct
Robin Rabenschlag, San Antonio, Texas

I got a call from a potential client, a 40 year old first mother, in her quest for natural birth. Roxanne told me that in her heart of hearts she wanted a home birth but her husband balked so she agreed to a hospital birth. Right away I had doubts as her doctor was not the most "natural" in delivery style. She also told me that her husband might be gone for seven days in her 38th week of pregnancy.

On her 38th week, I got a call from her saying that her water had broken. She told me that she wanted company. I left for her house so would she would have a continuous companion as her husband would not be back until later in the day.   I had serious doubts whether he would make it to the birth as her family history was filled with precipitous births.

When I got there she was not in any hurry to go to the hospital. She ate breakfast, worked on a school paper, called friends and took a long shower. By 1:30pm, she called the doctor's office and talked to an assistant who griped at her for not going to the hospital earlier. Her response to the woman on the phone was "I'm not having good contractions and I'm not coming now." She did get everything ready that she wanted to have at the hospital and finally acquiesced to go to the hospital later in the afternoon.

When we arrived in the labor and delivery unit, I breathed a sigh of relief as I found that my favorite obstetrician was on call and I knew my client's chances for a natural birth had grown tremendously.   The afternoon dragged on with not many contractions until the time her husband was supposed to arrive in town. Then her contractions became really uncomfortable but she said that she didn't want to move around until he got there.

He was a hour late and Roxanne was so happy to see him. I let them have some time alone and when I returned they were snuggling in each other's arms, slow dancing to lovely music. It was a serene scene. They then commented that they wanted to work actively to get their baby born so she spent much of the next few hours on the "birth ball." Since she felt safe, the labor quickly seemed to progress. She got into a ritual breathing pattern while sitting on the ball. At 7:30 pm, Roxanne asked to be checked and was 3-4 centimeters, 100% effaced and the baby was at a zero station. I suggested many labor support techniques. She changed positions often, alternating between leaning on the bed, walking in the room, slow dancing and kneeling over the birth ball. There was no IV in place and no continuous fetal monitoring and by 9:15 pm she was 5-6 centimeters. My relationship with the obstetrician helped as she trusted me to let the nurses know if we needed anything.

By this time, Roxanne decided to get in the shower and both her husband and I got quite wet assisting her. She was slowly turning inside herself during contractions but was quite witty and cheerful between them.   After her shower, she got back on the birth ball and the contractions were now tough for her to handle.

Shortly after 10 pm, she crawled up onto the bed on her side and began to make grunting noises. She started a "birth song" and her rituals were instinctual. She insisted that both her husband and I talk to her continuously. Next, she wanted to hear only MY voice.   My monotone noises were the longest, non-stop performance of guided imagery that I had ever done. Her husband held her hand, but all in the room except me, were totally quiet. I was kneeling on the floor very close to Roxanne as I guided Roxanne though the contractions verbally. I cradled her head in my arms and held her hand. The doctor nodded her head intermittently to let me know that everything was progressing normally and, in a few minutes, Roxanne's beautiful little boy glided out of her with the grace and ease of a quietly birthing animal in the peacefulness of its nest.

When the nurse took pictures of the birth, the reality hit Roxanne that she had given birth. She swept him up onto her belly and no one uttered a single tone or touched the baby except the mom and dad. It was so peaceful in the room. If I had I not looked around the room in the hospital, I would've sworn that we had stayed at home. She essentially got her longed for home birth in a hospital setting.

Even though this birth happened in a hospital that did more than 900 births a month, this experience proved to me that birth can be beautiful and serene if all in the room believe in birth. The nurse and doctor were enthralled in this natural event. This birth showed that birth was about family, love, and respect.

Sharing the Triumph
Joni Nichols, Guadalajara, Mexico

I worked for three years in a unpersonalized regional hospital located in the city center. I happened to be certified as both a childbirth educator and as a doula but in this environment, I believe that ANY warm body that could offer a smile of encouragement, an empathetic gesture, a gentle touch, or a soft word would elicit what the researchers noted in their observations.

My "gordas" (a Spanish affectionate word I use for pregnant women) labored barefoot in a large communal room wearing gowns that often had no ties and in beds that were little more than a metal frame and a two inch mattress. They had no access to food or water and their only sense of time was measured by the sunlight filtering in the few windows and the changing of the staff at 12 hour intervals. Upon being admitted into the hospital, the women entered alone and exchanged their possessions for a hospital issued gown that was often frayed, stained and too small. Not only did they leave their loved ones at the threshold but their personal identity as well.

I rarely met the ladies before labor, had sketchy information on their charts to go by, had little time to earn their trust and was handicapped by my foreign accent, but I knew that I could make a huge difference in their births. I acknowledged the woman's name, offered her a piece of adhesive tape to close her gown, offered a hand to hold, murmured words of encouragement, acted as a shield for the disapproval evident in the staff's faces when she strayed from the bed, and walked beside her proudly. The room was filled with clattering trays and instruments, the radio blaring songs, the cries from other birth women reverberating off the tiled floors, and the sounds of nervous pediatric residents who were anxiously hovering at the doctor's shoulder, ready to whisk the baby off to the nursery. Everybody except the doula and the laboring woman was hidden behind a mask. The more helpful nurses would at least cajole the women to push, the insolent ones would only stand by in silent disgust. The instructions by the resident doctor were mechanical and intoned with boredom. The pregnant women were essentially voiceless, nameless, and powerless. I thought the attention of a doula in that heartless, bureaucratic, and routinized setting of a public institution where there were no birthing choices, came closest to mothering the mother as the research indicated. The doula's presence was a powerful antidote to despair and loneliness. Over and over again, the value of "being there" was reaffirmed for me.

What I wore, what I charted, what position was used, which breathing pattern was employed, which trade secrets came in handy, paled beside the simple fact that someone honored the woman for giving birth to her child.

When I shared the triumph of birth with these women, memories were engraved in my heart forever.

A Hard, Prodromal Labor
Robyn Mattox,, Orlando, Florida

On December 30, I got a call from Sheri, a friend/client of mine telling me that she thought she was in labor. Sheri and I were pregnant together and my baby was a week overdue. Wow, she was going to have her baby before I was! Even though Sheri's contractions were painful and irregular, she asked me to come to her house. On arriving at the house, my assessment was that she was handling the contractions quite well. She remarked that her back hurt, so I suggested that she get in the hands-and-knees position over the birth ball while I did the hip squeeze technique. By 8pm, her intense contractions were 3 minutes apart so we headed to the birth center.

After the midwife's exam, she told us that Sheri was 2 centimeters dilated. We labored in the lounge watching TV while Sheri sat on the oval egg ball and her fiancee, Joe, massaged her back. Soon she was vocalizing through each contraction. After a hour, the midwife checked her again and her dilatation was 3 cm. After a few more hours, the midwife checked her again and told us that she was 4 cm. Throughout the night, Sheri was in and out of the tub and the back labor was taking a toll on her. She and Joe worked well together and the picture of him pouring water over Sheri's body while talking softly to her was an awesome sight.

By morning, Sheri was 5 centimeters and she was losing confidence. The back labor was getting worse and nothing seemed to be helping. The was a lull in the contractions for about a hour and that helped Sheri get a second wind. The midwife suggested a walk outside and off we went. The walk helped lift her spirits but no amount of counterpressure helped. After the next check, the midwife proclaimed "5 centimeters" and Sheri broke down crying. She asked for a drug to help her relax and received Nubain. By 1pm, I had to go home and let my pregnant body have some sleep. About 4pm, I got a phone call saying that Sheri was very upset and had told everyone to leave.

I came back to the birth center and Sheri was in a room by herself, allowing no one to come near her. I went in quietly and sat down in front of her. I didn't know what to do. I had tried all of my "doula tricks" and I was out of ideas. I said that she was doing wonderfully and asked how I could help her. She looked at me and asked "Do you think I should go to the hospital?" I told her that I couldn't tell her what to do, but we should talk about all of her options. I went over everything but mostly I listened and let her talk so that she could come to terms with what was happening. She asked if it was OK to go to the hospital. I could see that she wasn't asking my permission but was asking if I felt she had failed if she went to the hospital. Again, I told her that she hadn't failed and was a strong woman.

We made the transport to the hospital. We had to go through the business office to register and while there Sheri had a strong contraction, vocalizing through it like she had been doing at the birth center. The lady in admitting was frightened and didn't know what to do. Every nurse from anywhere around this office came running!

Ron was our labor and delivery nurse and I had worked with him before. When doing his assessment, he remarked that the baby was not only posterior but asynclitic. Once again, I talked with Sheri and Joe about options and she chose a walking epidural for pain relief. After the epidural, Sheri was almost back to her old self and tried the birth ball and other position changes. Pitocin was started in hopes of managing her dysfunctional labor pattern, and by 11pm, she was 8 centimeters. The nurse manager came in and asked Sheri and Joe if they would allow an interview if her baby was the first baby of the new millennium in this hospital. She noticed that I was large with child and asked when the baby was due. I told her then that my due date was last week but that my baby didn't understand due dates. Sheri was started joking about my rapid labors and that if I went into labor my home birth might be an "accidental" hospital birth.

At 1am, Sheri started pushing and by 2am she didn't made any progress and was exhausted. We were told that another hour was all we had until a cesarean would be ordered. Sheri did make progress but the resident came in to discuss forceps or a vacuum extraction. Joe and Sheri asked for more time and were told the resident would return in 20 minutes. The doctors hadn't been gone 30 seconds when Sheri exclaimed that the baby was coming down and the nurses scrambled to find a doctor. The doctor told Sheri she needed an episiotomy . I asked if she could try one or two more pushes before that was done and Joe re-iterated that Sheri did not want one by literally stopping the doctor with his hands. The doctor agreed to let her push a couple more times. With the next push, Sheri pushed the baby's head out and, within minutes, he was crying. Sheri was overwhelmed and Joe and I were crying like the baby was! The doctor had to leave for a few minutes to take care of an emergency. The supervisor walked in with another doctor and started telling Sheri about the vacuum extraction that she was doing to do. She was startled when she heard a baby cry and looked up and saw the baby in the warmer. So much for talking about vacuum extraction!

I went home very happy and tired. This was one of the hardest and longest births I had worked with. I went over everything in my mind that had happened for the last 48 hours. Could I have noticed the posterior position sooner? Was there anything else I could have done? When I saw Sheri the next day, it was rewarding to hear her say that just my presence and confidence in her, gave her the strength she needed to give birth.

I became a doula to make a difference in women's births. I can't always change the circumstances, but I can have a profound effect on the memory that the parent will carry with them for the rest of their life.

I was so glad that my own baby waited three more days to be born. It was almost as if the my baby knew that he needed to wait until Sheri's baby was born. Smart baby, my little Christopher!

We Do Make a Difference
Karen Kilson, Sandy Hook, Connecticut

My pager sounded at 8:15 am Tuesday, calling me to assist Molly in her labor. I arrived to find Molly's membranes had spontaneously ruptured the night before, at 35 weeks into her pregnancy. She was only in prodromal labor but was quite anxious, and when I sat down beside her, she relaxed visibly. I learned that Molly and Rick hadn't taken childbirth education classes and knew little about birth. Rick paced nervously. I answered their questions and gave them impromptu on-the-spot childbirth classes. By early evening, the plan was to move Molly to the maternity floor and let her sleep thought the night and then begin a pitocin induction in the morning. I went home to get a good night's sleep.

Bright and early in the morning, Rick called, asking me to be there for the initial pitocin dose. When I arrived at the hospital, I got to know them better and found that both of them had a wonderful sense of humor. For a few hours, Molly felt nothing uncomfortable and then began noticing when each contraction started. Together we breathed softly through them. There were many visitors in the room now and Molly had trouble concentrating. The resident noticed that and asked all to leave except Rick, Molly's dad , her aunt and me.

Time to get down to business. I got Molly out of the bed and showed Molly and Rick how to "slow dance" during contractions. Rick was way too nervous to do that, so I took his position in the labor support strategy. I gradually maneuvered Molly to rock with the "birth ball" next to the bed. This worked well and we continued breathing together. Soon, she announced that she felt low pressure in her pelvis.

The nurse checked Molly and said that she was 1 centimeter but the baby was very low in the pelvis. Molly was in and out of the bed for the next few hours. In my mind, I saw her as small doe looking for a safe place to birth her fawn. She worked well with her contractions but still seemed unsettled. I followed her lead and wherever she was, I was there massaging her. The next time the nurse checked, Molly was dilated to 3.5 centimeters, but Molly seemed to be disappointed with this news and got in the bed.

I thought that her family members might be helpful now. Molly was given Stadol and I lowered the lights in the room, positioned her family around her and put soft music on. Within minutes, her dad began stroking her head, her husband held her hand, her aunt stroked her arm, and I massaged her feet and legs. I gently encouraged her to loosen her muscles in her arms, legs, and jaw. Remembering the doe, I assured her that she was in a safe place with us and we would all stay with her. I asked her to look at the people surrounding her and feel their love and draw on their strength. The atmosphere in the room felt spiritual and I asked her to feel the warmth, security, and peace in the room.

On cue, Molly's contractions intensified and we again began actively helping her deal with them. She wanted total pain relief and asked for an epidural. The nurse began hydrating Molly by an IV, so she would be ready to receive an epidural. We were now working at full tilt and Molly needed to change positions every few minutes. Even Rick began talking to her through contractions to help her concentrate. Molly felt more pelvic pressure and when I asked her to not push during the contraction, she cried out "My body is doing it anyway." Only 90 minutes after the peaceful moments with her family, the nurse checked Molly at 4:10pm, and found she was completely dilated.

Rick stayed right close to her side and the second stage of her labor only lasted 30 minutes. Their 5 lb 4 oz little girl was born at 4:43pm, over an intact perineum, with Apgars of 9 and 9. Molly never had time to get the epidural. Molly and Rick spent some time with their little daughter before she had to go to the NICU for observation due to her prematurity. I went to the NICU and took an instant picture of her for her parents. Rick and others left to get food so I stayed with Molly. We talked about that spiritual moment when we all were around her bed. That was when she told me that she had "given herself permission" to go forward with the birth. When I left, I hugged her and expressed my pride in her for her strength and amazing labor work. Once again, I drove home feeling the amazing power of women, and being grateful to be able to work in a wonderful profession.

A Mother's Day Baby
Diane Tinker, Des Moines, Iowa

Due to an auto-immune disease, Sue had suffered several miscarriages since her first son was born nearly four years ago by cesarean. Sue told me that her doctor termed her "high-risk," but she was planning a VBAC with this pregnancy anyway. She and her husband researched the topic of VBAC thoroughly and felt that they needed a care provider who supported their decision to try for a vaginal birth this time. I supported them by listening to their frustrations. They had trouble finding a doctor that would take care of them due to the auto-immune disease and previous cesarean. They persisted and finally found a family practitioner who would take over her care. They wrote a birth plan that included plans for a cesarean birth if necessary. I worked with Sue and Bob on relaxation techniques and comfort measures.

I got a call one day saying that Sue was showing positive signs of early labor. This next day, Sue called and said that her water had just broken. I went to their home and found not only Sue and Bob and their son but many other family members as well. Sue was sitting on her birth ball. She and Bob decided to go for a walk in the park and I accompanied them. After the walk, she began to complain of back pain so I positioned her in the hands-and-knees position over the birth ball. Bob rubbed her back and applied counter pressure. Soon, Sue was exhibiting signs of transition, so the decision was made to go to the hospital.

When we arrived at the hospital, Sue was 6 centimeters. Sue and Bob were thrilled with her progress and, in no time, Sue was feeling an urge to push. The nurse checked, and Sue was still 6 cm, so Bob and I continued our routine of applying counter pressure and hot packs to her back. I talked to her through each contraction and she was coping well with the labor. By then it was midnight, and the thought occurred to me that it was now Mother's Day and I exclaimed to Sue, "You will be having the best Mother's Day gift- a baby."

With an increased urge to push, the nurse checked Sue again, and told her that she only had a rim of cervix left. Bob and I worked as a team. Sue's contractions became more intense and she no longer could resist the urge to push. The lip of cervix remained and when the nurse pushed it back over the baby's head it came right back. Sue was allowed to push for 1 ½ hours but to no avail. The doctor was very patient and told Sue she was pushing well but the baby wasn't moving down in the pelvis.

Sue was getting tired of the back pain but was strong and determined to birth her daughter vaginally. Suddenly, the baby's heart rate dipped into the 70's and was slow to come back up. The doctor told Sue not to push and an internal monitor was attached to the baby's scalp. Sue was allowed to push again but the baby was not moving down further. After no progress in descent, and a sudden, drastic rise in the baby's heart rate to the 190's, a decision was made by Sue, Bob and the doctor to do a cesarean. When Bob heard the doctor say " cesarean," he began to weep. I comforted him and told him that Sue was OK with the decision and the baby needed to be born. Sue was prepped for surgery and soon Bob and I were wheeling her to the OR.

The doctor agreed to let both of us in the OR. The doctor knew how hard Sue and Bob had worked to accomplish their goal of a vaginal birth and was very accommodating and respectful of their wishes for me to be present at the birth. The OR crew was taken back. Later, I found out that this hospital had never had a doula at a cesarean, or more than one person in the OR.

The experience in the OR was quite uplifting, as the anesthesiologist tried to make the birth memory a good one. He touched Sue's face when he talked to her, asked if she had any questions, put soft music on the radio, and when the baby was delivered put her where Sue could see her. Bob was in such awe that he couldn't videotape any longer so the anesthesiologist took over that task. He walked over by Sue and squatted down so that she that he could photograph from her viewpoint. I took still photographs for them too.

After the birth, Sue kept saying how happy she was and that she had not regrets. The baby was placed close to Sue and her hand was unstrapped so that she could touch her. All of that time, the baby was wide-eyed and looking at her momma. Bob was allowed to take his daughter to the nursery. Before he left, the doctor asked the OR and recovery room staff to return the baby to Sue in the recovery room. They said it had never been done before, but they would do it. Little Willow was back with Bob in about ten minutes. Sue began nursing immediately and I watched with joy as the bond was being indelibly formed between mother and daughter. It was an incredible feeling to know that this cesarean birth was such a positive experience for the family. They had so many regrets from their first cesarean, but this birth was different.

As I drove home that Mother's Day morning, I thought about how all of the staff worked so hard to made Sue and Bob's birth memory a wonderful one. I was glad that I was able to be a part of this exceptional Mother's Day memory.

Learning from a Birth

Crystal Sada, Mt. Holly, New Jersey

Even though I am a seasoned doula I'm amazed how, at every birth, I learn something new. Sometimes I learn about the process of birth. Sometimes I learn about women and their strength. Sometimes I learn about the professionals who care for women. Sometimes I learn about being a doula. This birth showed me that I had a preconceived prejudice that I didn't know existed.

A prospective client called and wanted to meet me. During the conversation, I discovered that her husband wanted nothing to do with having a doula at the birth. He felt that my presence would be a intrusion and that he could help her though the labor by himself. I explained that I had a strict policy about meeting whomever the primary support person would be. She said that she would talk to him and see if he would meet me. We talked several times throughout the next two weeks but he wouldn't budge about a meeting with a doula.

Then one evening, she called and said that her husband would meet with me for ONLY one hour. The following week we met. Without saying a word to him about his reluctance, I started talking as I usually do in a initial meeting. When the meeting was over, I realized that we had just talked for three hours. I apologized for going over the hour mark, but he spoke up and thanked me, saying that he had learned more in that three hours than he did in their whole childbirth class series. A few days later, I was hired to be their doula.

Five days after her due date, my client called and said she had been cramping all day at work and after lunch it got worse. I advised her to take a nice warm bath or shower and lay down. As I was hanging up, she stated that the fluid leaking was the worst part. Fluid, what fluid? I advised her to call her doctor. Then she told me her doctor was in another city right now.

About two hours later, I got a frantic phone call from the dad telling me to come NOW as his wife was 5 centimeters dilated. What?!! I grabbed my gear and left immediately. By the time I got to the hospital, she was 7 centimeters and the dad was doing a very good job of supporting her. Her wish was to deliver without drugs or interventions. I settled in and watched the two of them work. Every once in a while, the dad would look up at me, and I would give him the thumbs up or okay sign or give a suggestion.

After I had been there thirty minutes, I discovered that her doctor would not be at the delivery, and the doctor on call was a perinatologist. Immediately, I was somewhat concerned as my client had never met him AND he was a perinatologist! To me that spelled disaster. Most perinatologists that I had worked with in the past, were interventionists in a big way. They felt that labor was a accident waiting to happen and they were the cure.

By the time the doctor arrived, my client was 9 centimeters and feeling pushy. This doctor was a quiet man and seemed genuinely concerned that my client had never met him. He asked her how she felt about that. She basically said that if he could catch the baby she didn't care. We all laughed and that broke the ice. Soon my client was pushing in earnest. After the doctor examined her, he remarked that the baby was in an asynclitic position. I spoke up and asked if he knew how to fix that. He said "Yes" but it would hurt the client, and he would rather see if the mom could fix it herself. He suggested that she should push in the hands-and-knees position. Did my ears deceive me or did a perinatologist really say that? I was thrilled. After thirty minutes, the doctor came back and did a check again. Still the position remained the same. I suggested the stomp-squat technique but my client felt that she couldn't do that as she had already been pushing for three hours. I asked again if the doctor could fix the position. Again, he said it would hurt. I commented that may be true, but so would a cesarean and wasn't that were she was heading? So, without further debate, he reached up and turned the baby.

Then he did something that I had never seen before. He fashioned a little pool out of a plastic drape and got the nurse to pour warm water into the little pool at the end of the bed. For the life of me, I couldn't figure out what he was doing, and I was so intent on watching that I didn't ask. As my client pushed her baby out, the doctor guided the baby into the little pool and asked the mother to reach down and splash the water onto the baby and then pull her baby up to her. At first, she was afraid that she would drop the baby. He told her that he could drop baby, or maybe the nurse could drop the baby, but the mother would NOT drop her baby. This was truly one of the most empowering experiences I had been a part of. Afterwards, I asked the doctor if he did that all the time, and he said he did, as he felt the baby's transition into the world was easier this way. It was true as the baby hardly cried at all. This scene reminded me of the Leboyer births that we did in the late 70's and early 80's.

After the birth when I was getting my gear together and thinking about what I had done in the birth it dawned on me that the answer was almost nothing at all. Then I felt a presence over me and turned to find the dad standing over me. He gave me a bear hug and said he couldn't have done it without me, as he didn't know how intense labor could be. I told him I was quite impressed with the care he care to his wife. He then said that every time he looked at me and I gave him the thumbs up sign, he knew that everything was going just as it should. He had learned that doulas were for both the mother *and* the father. This birth convinced him to be a true supporter of doulas!

This birth taught *me* two things. Don't be judgmental or have preconceived ideas about medical professionals. Sometimes the only things you need in your doula bag is your thumbs, a smile, and a loving heart.

A Unfilled Dream
Teri Gulker

I had a nurse-friend who went to a seminar where Polly Perez was speaking and mentioned the work of the doula. She immediately got the book, *Special Women,* and was so excited that it was signed by the author herself. She used the information in the book in her work as a labor and delivery nurse with her patients- massaging them, teaching them labor support techniques, and believing in their ability to birth their baby. She would work circles about me and she was the reason that I learned to love OB. Carol so much wanted to be a doula. She was compassionate, encouraging, and giving to her patients and to her colleagues .

Two years after I started working with Carol, she was diagnosed with cancer. Soon it was clear that the cancer had spread but Carol kept working with birthing women. She loved to help women give birth and enjoyed the delivery process so. She was such an advocate for women! She still had a dream about being a doula. She put her heart and soul in her work and continued working until the last two weeks before she died.

Carol was a truly special woman in my life. After her death, I so wanted to have something of hers, to remind me of her and her dream. That was when I found her autographed copy of *Special Women* outlining the traits of a doula: professional, enthusiastic, a clear thinker, tactful, patient, resilient, strives for excellence, a good listener, progressive thinker, and a "special woman." It described my friend Carol perfectly.

...through the eyes of mothers and labor assistants

Not What I Planned
Stephanie Soderblom, the mother, from Denver, Colorado

I am a doula myself and when I planned the birth of my second child I hired TWO doulas to attend my longed for home birth. I chose each doula after a lot of careful thought as to what exactly I was going to expect of my doulas. The first one, Cobie, was a good friend of mine and who has a loving, soft side to her that was unsurpassed by anyone I have ever met. She was the type of person that made you feel nurtured.....but I knew that I also needed a strong and assertive hand. Kim was to be my second doula, and the one that I could draw on when I felt that I had no strength left inside of me.

As my due date came and went, I began calling on my doulas for encouragement but it wasn't until my water broke that they would prove just how valuable a professional labor assistant can be. My heart sank when my water broke, as I knew before I hired Cobie, there was one weekend that she would not in town. It was this weekend.

When I called Kim she came right over. She massaged my feet while we talked. I felt very nurtured but I had an internal feeling that something was wrong. I began to say this out loud, complaining that something wasn't right. Thirteen hours after my membranes ruptured I was only 2-3 centimeters.

Everyone was exhausted but Kim stayed with me while the others went to bed. Night can be a scary time when you are in labor but I wasn't alone. She laid in my bed with me and I found comfort in her presence. By morning, the contractions was almost stopped and I begged Kim to go home as nothing was happening. That night I asked everybody to go to sleep.

About 11:30pm, the contractions started again with a vengeance. In about fifteen minutes, they went from tolerable, mild contractions to ones where I doubled up saying "help me." My husband begged me to let him call Kim. I said NO. She had been there so long and I didn't want to bother her until I was sure I was really in labor. My husband told me that he needed Kim for HIM so her called her to come back anyway.

When Kim arrived she immediately held my hand and began saying soothing words in my ear. She sat by my side, stroked my hair, and reminded me to relax my legs and shoulders. I kept saying to anyone that would listen "Something is wrong as this doesn't feel right." I began complaining about by bladder and was worried that I had a bladder infection.

Cobie drove all night to get home to me and she arrived about 4:30am. For the next few hours, both of my professional birth assistants walked with me. I started talking with then and my midwife about going to the hospital. I knew something was wrong. At 5:30am, I announced, "We need to leave for the hospital as this is not right." We loaded up and drove to the hospital were I screamed that I had a bladder infection and needed help.

The assessment showed that I did have a bladder infection and a temperature of 100.7degrees F. The baby began passing meconium and her heart rate was fast. Before long, I was hooked up to an IV, an epidural, amniofusion, internal fetal monitor and internal pressure monitor, Foley catheter, and pitocin........everything I had hoped to avoid. My fever climbed to 102.7 when the decision to have a cesarean was made. I was heart broken. My labor assistants and I cried from frustration.

I hugged my labor assistants on the way to the OR where my healthy baby girl was born at 12:37pm. Having professional labor assistants at my birth let me know first hand how little touches can make a difference to not only to me but to my husband as well.

Kim, the doula, Denver, Colorado

Stephanie and I were in the same doula training class and I was so honored to be part of her birth. I got a call from Stephanie while I was grocery shopping with my children and had to leave the store to call her back. I clearly remember standing in the rain talking on the phone to her while my children were pushing their Customer-in-Training carts around and wondered if they would be able to finish their shopping experience.

Stephanie told me that her water had broken and her contractions were mild but she wanted to give me a "heads up" sign because she felt that she would need my support soon. The kids and I rushed through our shopping trip.

In about an hour, she called again and I left for her house which is about one hour away. When I got there, I spent time massaging her feet and hands and also applying pressure to acupressure points that would help speed her labor. She was in high spirits and changed her position from sitting in a recliner to sitting on the birth ball. As the afternoon progressed, her contractions began to intensify. I walked with her and we changed the scenery by moving to the porch, even though it was still raining. I held Stephanie through a long contraction as the rain came gently down.

I helped by going to the health food store to get Echinacea tincture to help prevent infection for Stephanie. I took advantage of the trip to the store to eat, as I knew it might be a long night and I needed to keep my energy up. It seems that Stephanie had an unremitting pain in her lower pelvis between contractions. As the evening got later, she was disheartened and needed encouragement from both her husband and me. Her contractions were on top of each other and she was beginning to feel a lot of pelvic pressure.

The midwife checked Stephanie's progress and told us that she was 2 cm and 80% effaced. I was mystified, as I usually could tell the mother's progress by her behavioral changes. I thought Stephanie would have been 5 cm or so. Disappointment invaded the room and

Stephanie cried and cried. All of us encouraged her and finally her mood seemed to lighten. The midwife gave her some herbs to help her relax and then left again. I was surprised as I thought that midwives stayed continuously and provided doula-like support. Stephanie and Brian went to their bedroom to rest so I laid down on the couch and slept for three hours. Not much was happening but the pelvis pain was still there. Stephanie asked me to go home for awhile.

I spent the day with my husband and children but I was worried that I hadn't heard from Stephanie. I was concerned about infection. I awakened to the phone ringing. It was Brian telling me that he had checked Stephanie and she was 3 cm and the contractions were intense. He said I should come. When I got there, Stephanie was in the portable tub and her contractions were 2 minutes and lasting 60-90 seconds. Her baby writhed as each contraction washed over her. I desperately wanted to take the pain away from Stephanie but instead I held her and encouraged her. Cobie arrived and the midwife came back and found the Stephanie was 3cm but her cervix was swelling. For another hour, Stephanie was back in the labor pool and nothing seemed to be helping her. At 4:37am, the decision was made to transport to the hospital. We made the trip to Boulder Community Hospital as it supported home birth and lay midwives. I kept thinking what else I could have done to help her have her longed for home birth.

When we arrived at the hospital, Stephanie stood up and pea soup meconium poured out of her vagina. At that point, I had to leave for a moment to so that I could release varied emotions- worry, fear and disappointment. Many interventions followed including an epidural. I was asked to take the midwife to her car and I didn't feel good about leaving Stephanie and Brian. I was told that nothing would happen until the doctor came back at 11am. I had a sense of foreboding. This was one of those moments that I haven't forgiven myself for yet. I knew better than to leave. I should have trusted my instincts. When I arrived back at the hospital, I saw Stephanie being wheeled out into the hall. No words needed to be spoken as I knew what that meant. For a brief moment, I held Stephanie and we cried together. She had been though so much and wanted a cesarean least of all. I was heartbroken for her. I was emotionally and physically wasted and spent 10 minutes crying. Finally, Brian came out with a beautiful baby girl named Kerstyn. I cried again as she was so wondrous and healthy. It was such a miracle.

I saw Stephanie in the recovery room and held her hand. Soon she was wheeled to the nursery where she got to hold her little daughter. Seeing mother and daughter gaze at each other, was a beautiful sight to behold.

The Birth of Clare Elizabeth

Deb Sexton, the mother, from Normal, Illinois

Our dream baby, Clare Elizabeth, was born on August 26, 1986. What made this birth unique for me was the fact that we had had three children born by Cesarean sections. Clare was a carefully planned and longed for VBAC (vaginal birth after cesarean) baby. With the help of our doula, Sue Frizzell, we were able to do much reading about VBAC and natural birth. Sue did the footwork in finding answers to my questions, locating medical articles, and loaning us books and pamphlets. She accompanied me to prenatal visits with my obstetrician. She followed up with information on routine procedures he recommended. Sue enabled us to make informed choices and I felt confident in refusing some of those procedures.

Sue helped me in so many other ways. She never doubted that our VBAC would be successful and her nurturing, loving, and caring ways gave me the support I needed through pregnancy and labor. She had me write down what I ate so we could make sure I was well-nourished. She provided me with herbs for tea that I enjoyed greatly.

On the Sunday before Clare was born, I began having contractions twenty minutes apart. My husband, Tim, was working and I knew it was too early to call Sue so I went about doing everyday things and got through the contractions alone.

On Monday, with Tim, our other children, Sue and our friend Julie present the atmosphere was comfortable and low-key. A local midwife, Betty, came to help monitor labor later in the day. As labor progressed it was clear to me that this baby could be born at home but we had not prepared for a home birth. At my husband's insistence we made the trip to the hospital.

It certainly was a different atmosphere at the hospital--lots of lights, people, noise and activity. Labor progressed somewhat slowly there. I was able to use the squat bar on the birthing bed and I continued to drink and eat lightly. Sue had given me a homemade recipe for laborade (an electrolyte-balanced lemonade) that I drank. I also had plain yogurt and orange juice popsicles.

I am so thankful for my birth team. As the birth work got harder and harder, I sensed that Sue was focusing more and more on me. She reminded me to chant in a low voice. She encouraged me to repeat the affirmations I used before labor to remind me of my inner power. As I grew more and more tired, Sue helped me maintain positive emotional and psychological energy. She helped me relax. She did massage. She seemed to rely on her birthing instincts. Tim was holding my face in his hands and helping me concentrate and I needed him to stay there. I did not want him out of my sight. He was my loving focus. Even when I could not talk, Julie seemed to understand when I needed bites of popsicle or sips of laborade. Thanks to her we also have lovely birth photos.

I can hardly describe the joy and love I felt as Clare came out of my body after two hours of pushing. After three cesarean births, I had pushed out my own baby. Nothing could diminish my feelings about Clare and her birth, not even the internal monitor or the episiotomy. I remember saying "my dream baby" over and over. And she truly was. All the love, support, nurturing and positive attitudes of my birth team had helped me reach that point of fulfillment.

Deb's Birthing of Clare
Sue Frizzell, doula

When Deb asked me to be her doula, I was thrilled! Like so many other birth attendants, I love what I do. I knew this birth would be one of especially strong energy and beauty because of Deb. I felt she had grown alot psychologically and the icing on the   cake--so to speak--would be this VBAC. This VBAC after three cesareans was to be VIP (Very Important Politically) too.

Deb and Tim met with our local midwife, Betty, who had agreed to be the primary monitrice for the home labor before their planned hospital birthing room birth. As her due date came and went, Deb had a lot of warm-up contractions. When labor finally started and she called me to attend her. I listened to fetal heart tones, kept labor notes, and saw that she ate, drank and rested. Her husband was with her as was a close friend, Julie. We all shared the duty of being a companion to her other three children, Emily, Tyler, and Sarah. Later in the evening when labor seemed to be progressing, Betty came to help.

It was a calm, warm night, with good feelings all around. Deb labored in the timeless way of all women, following her body's rhythms. As the labor progressed the one thing that I was not prepared for was Deb desiring to birth at home. After discussing the issues and feelings it was clear that Tim still felt the need to go to the hospital for the birth, so we kept to our original plan. While Tim drove, I helped Deb breathe through contractions. I tried to help her continue to feel nurtured during this transport because I knew this was a very vulnerable time.

When we arrived at the hospital, I remembered the wise words of the midwife who had attended me at my birth. She said "see that there is a good emotional atmosphere, good consistent monitoring, and simple teamwork." Unfortunately, the very first contact with hospital personnel was a nurse with an extremely negative attitude. The three of us tried to insulate Deb from this. We were pleased when a friend of ours, who was on the staff dropped in. Then the head nurse, who was very nice, came to be our labor nurse. To help cultivate the sense of teamwork, I gave her a lot of strokes.

In helping Deb, I drew most, as I always do, from my own good, natural birth experience and from things I had learned from my midwife. The basics never change. As Deb labored, I used my intuition and observation to figure out how to help her. I stroked her face and shoulders when she seemed tense. I made low sounds to remind her to keep her own voice low and let the birth energy down and out. I knew that "open mouth--open bottom" was an important concept to all births. I helped her remain confident by reminding her of her chosen birth affirmations. As she squatted during the second stage, I remembered my own birth and was aware of the incredible energy going through her and her babe.

This birth was the first time I had ever acted as a doula in the hospital and I learned a few things that could be helpful to others. There might be uncertainty about what other people are thinking or what they will do next. I learned that openness and total focus on each birth is not the style in institutional settings. It is more difficult to keep the birthing energy totally focused and centered in the hospital than at home or in a birth center. I did wish afterward that when interventions were suggested I had thought to ask, "would you like time to think about things?"

I had thought they would rush Clare away to be suctioned due to the meconium, so I was determined to help Deb touch her immediately as she emerged. Her touch was electric and I still remember Deb's cry, "My baby!" I was pleasantly surprised that they used only the bulb syringe to suction the baby and never took her from her mama's arms.

My favorite images of the birth are those of Tim and Deb, head to head, with him holding her while she squatted on the bed during the second stage. This labor helped them bond to each other as they supported each other and shared the labor. I felt a sense of wonder at Clare who seemed wiser than any of us there. I felt privileged to have been asked to attend them on this powerful journey.

Home Birth/Transport/Cesarean Birth
Connie Banack, the mother, Camrose, Alberta, Canada

This was to be my first home birth after two hospital births, both ending in cesareans for failure to progress. Two days past my due date, I was having consistent contractions but they weren't painful so I went to bed. In the middle of the night, I was awoken by a contraction and alternated sitting on the birth ball or leaning on a pillow on the kitchen table while sitting on the birth ball. I called my doula and she arrived right before my husband woke up to go to work. Of course, he stayed home. Tracy used the Flax-Rap on my back while she applied counter pressure as I had back pain. My midwife arrived mid-morning and said that I was 2-3 centimeters dilated. I was concerned about the baby's position as my first two babies were posterior but the midwife said this baby was in a left occiput position. My contractions were getting increasingly stronger and longer, and I was having two contractions close together and then a break. I continued laboring though the day and used the birthing tub where Tracy pressed on my pelvis from each side. Running water on my back also helped. By 6 pm, I was almost completely dilated and my midwife decided to try to push the anterior lip back over the baby's head. OUCH!! It didn't work so I kept laboring in the tub and getting out to go to the bathroom. By 11pm, the lip was still not gone but the baby was at a + 2 station. The midwife tried once again to move the lip back...no luck.

By 2am, I was exhausted. The back up midwife had arrived. Tracy and Noreen tried to get some sleep while my husband and Barbara provided the counter pressure during contractions. All three of us slept in between contractions. The contractions kept double peaking and spaced out to 6 minutes. By morning, I was a bit refreshed and we tried one more time to push the lip back. We could move the lip back but the baby didn't move down anymore, so I sobbingly consented to transfer to the hospital.

Tracy was a constant emotional support as I mentally prepared for the cesarean I was facing. She was there to ensure that my birth plan was honored. She was not allowed into the OR with my husband so we compromised on my husband being there for the surgery/delivery and Tracy coming in when he left to go to the nursery. I was able to hold my newborn son after he was born. It was wonderful to have someone there constantly for me. Tracy watched the rest of the surgery and told me what they were doing and then went with me to the recovery room. I would never birth without a doula again. It made all of the difference in the world.

Tracey de Hoop, doula, Edmonton, Alberta, Canada

I was very excited when my sister asked me to be her doula for her third birth. When Connie called in labor, it was about 5 am and I had an hour drive to get to her home. When I arrived, she was laying cocooned in blankets in the front room as she didn't want to wake her husband. Soon Connie was walking around the house and the contractions became harder. The midwife was called and when she checked Connie I was glad to hear that she was 2-3 centimeters. I started helping Connie by doing many labor support techniques that ran the gamut from stair climbing to my version of the hip squeeze. Connie then got into the birthing pool and by early evening she was almost completely dilated. We continued laboring throughout the night.

The next morning, Connie started to push but the baby wouldn't budge. After much discussion with all involved in the birth, Connie and Allan decided to transport to the hospital. At the hospital, things started happening quickly so I tried to be sure that Connie's alternate birth plan was followed. I think that Connie was glad to have something happening after over 17 hours of intense back labour and more than 12 hours of no progress. A cesarean was decided on. I tried to get the staff to let both Allan and I accompany Connie to the OR but it was to no avail. I could hear my nephew, Brendan Connor Banack, cry from where I was outside of the OR. I started crying. knowing that he had finally arrived. I was able to go into the OR after the birth when Allan took the baby to the nursery, so Connie would not be alone.

When I got into the OR, I let Connie know what was happened in the surgery and tried to keep her warm as she was shivering . That was hard to do when you could only touch her hand and arm. This was one of the hardest births I had ever attended, and not because my sister had a cesarean that she didn't want, but because it was very, very hard for me to watch her go through so much pain. It was harder since she was not only my client, but my sister.

Birth: Two Perspectives

Carol Ritolo, the mother, from Toronto, Ontario, Canada

My first two babies were born by cesarean, both five weeks early. With the first my husband, Mark, and I knew very little, and did not try to avoid the cesarean, which was done for "fetal distress" at eight centimeters. Later I discovered that it may have been unnecessary so I changed doctors and planned a VBAC with my second. In labor we discovered the baby was in a transverse breech presentation, so I had another cesarean.

I felt okay about this cesarean. Everything had been explained to me and because I had already had a cesarean it didn't seem too shocking. Still, I felt cheated. I had done a lot more preparation, but I still didn't know about labour support.

Before I became pregnant again, I acquired more information. I learned a lot while training to be a prenatal teacher. I attended workshops with Nancy Cohen (a leader in the movement to lower the cesarean rate) and joined a VBAC support group. I began to question my doctor a lot. I presented him with a birth plan and he was very intimidated. He said that he was not sure whether he would let me have the baby vaginally. I was very angry. I cried and he seemed bothered by my reaction. He couldn't understand why it was important to me--he couldn't wait to get out of the room. Although I had really liked him, I switched doctors.

With this pregnancy I switched at six and a half months to a more supportive doctor and chose to have labour support. I feel support is half the battle--it can't all be on my husband's shoulders.

I went into labour around 9pm on August 11, but was unsure because I had had so much false labour and my due date was not until August 31. I worked around the house and told March not to rush home, but by 4:30am, it was pretty clear. I phoned Janice, arranged babysitting and headed for the hospital. When I arrived at 6am, I found that Janice had already admitted me--which made it much easier for us--all I had to do was sign in. A nice nurse admitted me and I put on my own nightie. Only one unsupportive person came in and I used body language to get rid of her.

I was in good humour until I lost control about 8:30 or 9am. I was tired and hungry. I didn't like being stuck in that room, not having anywhere else to walk. And I didn't want to be touched. I did alot of self-massage and I talked to the baby. Having "permission" from Janice to vocalize--rather than breathe--was good. I breathed my own way, *noisily*. Saying it hurt made me feel better. Screaming sometimes relieved the tension and sometimes intensified it.

I was screaming for medication and felt at that point that a cesarean was the easy way out. Although I begged for an epidural, Janice and March talked me out of it. They knew my pleas were really a cry for help. I couldn't be touched so talking was what kept me going. I was really tired. I needed encouragement, not drugs. I needed the doctor to say "This is where you are and you're doing OK." I wanted him to be there and I felt the staff was not getting him for me. I don't feel badly about asking for the medication. Even homebirthers have told me that there was a point where they wanted to quit and go to the hospital for an epidural.

The end of the labour was really intense. I changed from my own full length gown into a hospital johnnie. I should have brought a short, easily opened gown. When the doctor did arrive, it was a relief. I was six to seven centimeters dilated and he asked about breaking my waters and I didn't answer. I didn't want to make that decision. Once he did it, so much fluid came out I was glad he did it because it was probably holding me back. I jumped quickly to my feet and four or five contractions later I had to bear down. My whole body did it. I was overwhelmed by the urge--it was so strong! I hadn't expected that. The only way to deal with the urge is to do it. The doctor said there was a lip and he kept his hand inside to stretch me. He finally said to start pushing and the first couple of pushes were ineffective. I was grabbing my husband's arm above my head but the doctor advised him to support my feet. Pushing was a whole new experience. My labour support person was beside me, keeping me on track. In fact, everyone was helping. Once I was in tune, I found pushing quite harmonious and positive. I was no longer just having contractions with no idea of where I was. Other women say they felt their baby moving down but I didn't, so it made it harder. I was told to touch the baby's head. I didn't want to but once I did, I was excited to feel it right at the opening. Then I could hardly stop pushing as the doctor guided the head out. I was thrilled that I had done it, that it was another boy, that I had pushed the baby out, that *I had given birth.* I cried. I got to hold him first and stroked and talked to him. Eventually I nursed him.

Every woman in labour should have a knowledgeable woman there--labour support other than a husband/partner, no matter how supportive he is. As a teacher I learned alot. I had always thought the breathing was the be-all and end-all. Now I think it's a bunch of garbage. I'd rather stress relaxation, being active, trying new positions, but above all having an experienced person by you the whole time.

Janice Pearson, doula

I always feel ambivalent when I think about being with a labouring couple. I want to help. I know I have the personal skills they need. But I do hate the waiting and I worry about my stamina. I don't stay up long hours or miss meals normally and this makes me anxious. With this pregnancy I was ambivalent. I was never sure March wanted this pregnancy, so I feared his support would be affected. I often worried that Carol wanted this child because she so dearly wanted a vaginal birth and a daughter. But I also know that any woman deserves love and attention at her birthplace. I rejoiced when Carol switched doctors this time. I felt her other doctor was a fine technician but would not give Carol the support and emotional back-up she would need for this birth.

When the birth is a planned VBAC there are hurdles no one should face alone. One of these hurdles is the need for the mother to remain unmedicated. Despite Carol's knowledge she had not had an unmedicated labour, so I knew we would have to work hard to keep her to that goal. I do confess that I dreaded the possibility that this might be another cesarean, but I truly believed that, by working together we could all get the baby out vaginally and joyfully.

The first hour of Carol's labour was uneventful. She couldn't sit down or lie down and did not want to be touched at all. I didn't know what to do with myself. As her labour advanced, I reminded her to let go a bit. She had been very controlled and I felt some vocalization was a good idea. So Carol got quite noisy!

It was really tough when Carol started to hint, and then insist, that she have an epidural. Because I couldn't touch her and she was very angry, I had to meet that request with firmness. During contractions I encouraged, between I reasoned. Carol asked, then pleaded, then yelled, then sobbed. Sometimes I was very soft with her but she just got louder. She was doing well and I just kept telling her that.

When her doctor arrived, he was very positive with her for being seven centimeters dilated and suggested an amniotomy to speed up labor. This was even harder than Carol asking for the epidural. I knew she wanted no intervention but I trusted her doctor and I knew it was going to be really hard to keep her from going to medication soon. I listened to the long silence, then said that I felt Carol would agree if it meant avoiding a cesarean. I gave Carol a chance to disagree and she didn't.

Only a few contractions later Carol had the urge to push. There were a few more hairy contractions with a rim and Carol was screaming. Then we all encouraged her to push. It took only twenty five minutes and Carol was asking if there was a quicker way. I said yes and she didn't want it. Carol kept saying a cesarean was easier. It was pretty exhilarating when I saw the head and realized she was going to do it.

I feel her birth could have been quite different. Carol could easily have had an epidural. When she was begging for one, a nurse was standing by and I felt real antagonism--that she felt I was wrong for discouraging Carol from taking one. I felt she thought it was not my business to do so. What if I had not been there or Carol had not had the doctor who believed she could do it? What if the hospital staff had been more vocally opposed to what she was doing? I really don't know if Carol's own efforts would have been enough. That scares me. Although labour support does not get the baby born, it certainly seems to help it get born the way the mother wants. I'm very glad I was there.

Fast and Furious
Robyn Mattox, mother, Orlando, Florida

I was 41.5 weeks pregnant and I needed my midwife's approval to continue with my plans to birth at home. On my office visit she stripped my membranes and told me that I was already 4-5 centimeters dilated. The next morning I woke up with mild contractions about 2 minutes apart. At 8:20am, I decided to sit in the bath tub and as soon as I relaxed in the water my contractions picked up. At 9:20 am, I called my midwife and told her I was in labor. The contractions were much worse and seemed to be right on top of each other. Bill was busy getting the pool set up as I was planning a water birth. The kids were awake now and I was moaning loudly. Once the pool was filed, I got out of the tub and into the pool. That made a big difference as the water in the pool was much deeper and covered more of my body.

The contractions became overwhelming and when my labor assistant and photographer arrived I was almost screaming but trying to keep the tone low. My husband was sitting behind me in the pool rubbing my back and shoulders saying encouraging words. It was now 10am and I was telling myself that I couldn't do this anymore. Being a doula I knew the signs of transition and tried to convince myself that it would be over soon. Then I let out a large groan and my water broke. Immediately I felt the baby slip down into my pelvis. My labor assistant told me to open my eyes and look at her and then said "The baby is here." She reached down into the water and found the baby crowning. I pushed once and the baby slipped into the water and Kathy took the baby out of the water and put him on my chest. My husband grabbed the blanket and suctioned the baby's mouth and put a blanket over him.

I was overwhelmed and kept saying "OH MY GOD" over and over. Chris looked up at my husband and me, and just stared at us. He pinked up right away and never cried. About 10 minutes later, the midwife arrived just was I was ready to deliver the placenta. I got out of the pool and laid down and nursed Chris for the first time.

I still can't believe how fast the labor was: 2 hours and 49 minutes. It was very different having this baby at home. When I had my first two children I was in a hospital and had a epidural. It was nice not to have the external monitors around me. I would definitely do it again at home. It wasn't exactly what I imagined it would be like but the experience was a good one.

Kathy Bradley, professional labor assistant, Rockledge, Florida

My relationship with Robyn began almost three years before the birth of her baby when she trained to become a doula. Robyn was planning a home birth and hired me to be her professional labor assistant. I got the call that Robyn was in labor about 9:15 am and found that she had only been in labor for a hour but the contractions were 2-3 minutes apart. I quickly dressed and hit the road as it would take about 40 minutes to reach her house.

Upon entering the house I found that I had reached Robyn before the midwife. Robyn was in the birth pool looking like she was working hard. Her husband was beside the pool with his attention on Robyn. I squatted down close to Bill and gently said hello to them. Robyn began to cry and tell me how hard this was. I calmly reminded her that her last two babies where born under epidural anesthesia and these sensations were new to her. She had another contraction and was tensing her shoulders so I reminded her to "let go and let birth happen." I felt it wouldn't be long before the birth happened and asked the doula there to be sure that the "birth kit" was ready. When Robyn had the next contraction, her body instinctually began birthing this baby. I firmly told her to "Open her eyes and blow" but she only could say, "The baby is right there." I reached down into the water and felt the head crowning. I exclaimed to Robyn, "Breathe your baby out slowly," but the baby had other ideas and came shooting out into the birth pool. I lifted him onto Robyn's chest where she and Bill talked to and massaged him. We were all quite stunned. The baby was doing fine, so Robyn kept him warm on her chest and we waited for the midwife who came about 10 minutes later.

Usually I spend many hours with my clients but this time with a precipitous delivery I only sent five minutes doing labor support and instead I did "birth support." The outcome was wonderful and I had to remind myself that sometimes you have to run with the punches and enjoy the blessings.

...through the eyes of a father

Clive Pohl, a father, Seattle, Washington

Our first child was born at home seven weeks ago and, as might be expected, we've been falling in love with her more every day. She's a beauty!

However, we could not have known how her delivery, and my involvement in it, would unfold. Lissa and I, having taken six weeks of home birth classes (and having prepared psychologically for nine months), felt ready. We had prepared a birth plan, reviewed it with our midwife, vacuumed the bedroom(!), and even prepared for the possibility of a hospital visit.

Lissa went into labor at 8 o'clock on a Saturday evening and straight into contractions five minutes apart. I timed their duration and frequency and stayed by her full of anticipation and a little afraid, but determined to do as much as I could. At 11 pm our trusty midwife came and measured Lissa's dilation at 3 cm and graciously said, "Try to get some rest; I'll see you in the morning." Fat chance! We labored on, contractions 3 minutes apart and increasingly intense--we were sure the baby would come by morning. As the contractions intensified and I perceived Lissa turning inward my intensity increased.

"Look at me, Sweety, count my fingers: 4,3,2,1,ahhhhhh! 3,2,1, ahhhhhh! Look at me!"

Though I was concerned by her pain and feeling more helpless than ever, I was determined to breathe every breath and to take her pain on myself. Fact is, I was a little bit in her face (though, miraculously, she only snapped at me once through the entire labor!) when all she really needed at this early stage was my presence. As we would discover, the contractions would get worse.

At 9:30 am after all that work, our midwife came back with all of her professional calm and measured Lissa at just 3 and a half centimeters! So much for the baby coming before noon! Exhausted, I eventually disengaged myself and my intense coaching from Lissa (though I remained with her) as our midwife and our labor assistant coached her through each contraction. I sat back and watched and listened. Their calm and careful choice of words was incredible t me, and inspirational, after such an intense night.

Gently...

"Stay with it..ride the wave, Lissa, that's it."

"Remember, your cervix has never opened in 29 years! It should take a while!"

I relaxed and listened and learned from them. I could not take my love's pain away. I could not take it upon myself. It was her pain and that was the only way it could be.

We labored on and progressed slowly and, infact, I did eventually come back to that level of intense involvement, but only during those few contractions when I sensed her spirits were sinking--transition, I think! I offered encouragement and as much love as I could, but now without trying to take her pain away. She was doing it!

Then, after two hours of pushing, a much needed episiotomy, and an amazing display of reserve energy on Lissa's part, the baby was born at 7:49 that Sunday evening; 9 lb., 4 oz. and the most beautiful thing we'd ever seen!

After calmly and capably sewing Lissa up, thoroughly cleaning our baby and our house, our midwife, our assistant and the proud parents gathered by the bed and discussed the unfolding of this special day.

When and if we have a second child I will go into my wife's labor with some lessons learned and some other lessons still to learn.

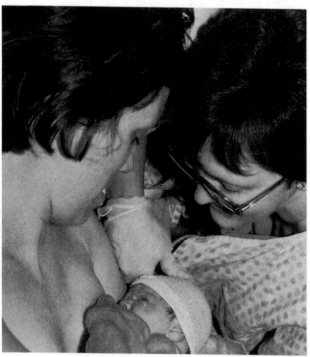

The need for support continues after
the birth of the baby

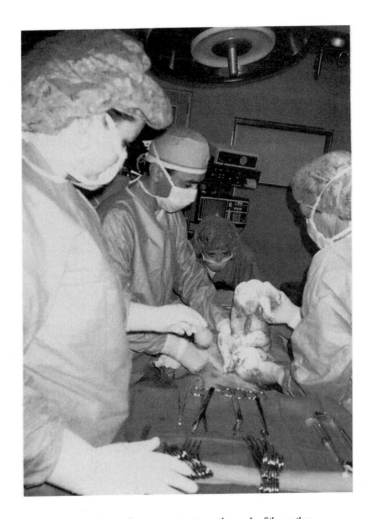

The labor assistant concentrates on the needs of the mother
during a cesarean birth.

12.
Afterword

Caring, Dignity, Courage, and Love

The earlier chapters of this book describe the role of the labor assistant with its joys and its drawbacks. As anyone can see, the role can be filled only by special women. This afterword summarizes these special women's desirable attributes. After reading this book, I hope some of you readers will count yourselves among these Special Women!

Labor assistants feel strongly that their contribution as a doula or monitrice is helping to change the way maternity care is provided in their area. They want and need to feel their contribution is making a difference. They often see themselves as the guardians of normal birth. They want women's choices about their birth to be respected. They want to help women grow and experience a joy they have never known before. They fully realize the impact the birth experience can have on women's lives and want the impact to be positive.

Most doulas or monitrices love birth and have a strong desire to help influence the beginning of life. One doula explains her feelings about her role by saying, "I wanted to do something important in a real sense; I want to know that my life counts. I really want to help others."

The rewards from this intense, demanding role are great. The relationships established with clients extend far beyond the actual birth. Many labor assistants find their clients often become their close friends because they have shared a time that will bond them together for many years to come.

The labor assistant often leaves the birth with the knowledge that she her presence helped the parents have the type of birth they wanted instead of a "routine" experience. She has a wonderful feeling of knowing that she empowered those in her care.

"My labor assistant made me feel strong, as if I were just a seedling before. Now I am an oak and my roots are firmly attached, nothing can sway me from my place of strength."

The labor assistant gains much from seeing others take responsibility for themselves, their birth, and their baby. The strength the family gains during this experience often influences the family members for the rest of their lives. It is a proud feeling for her to know that she has helped bring humanity and kindness back to the birthing process; to know that her presence helped ensure that this family was treated with the respect it deserved. It is a peaceful feeling to know that she has helped a couple feel comfortable medically and emotionally; to know she helped them to have a natural birth.

Since this job requires many and varied skills, the labor assistant must be a jack of all trades. She must demonstrate loyalty to her clients while trying to interface with hospital personnel. She may often be called upon to interpret what others have said. She has to be able to explain to others in the maternity care field how her work benefits her client, the baby, and the birth. She is politically aware. She shares credit for her accomplishments through helping others accept those accomplishments more easily.

She is a professional. She must be accountable for her actions. She must understand the big picture; she must be able to see how birth fits into not only each client's life and also the client's loved ones. She must constantly update her skills in order to help those in her care. She must always strive for excellence in her work; her work must be thorough.

She must be available around the clock and prepared to adjust her priorities when a mother calls reporting that she is in labor. She must have developed good listening skills and the ability to answer questions in a clear, concise manner. She must respect each mother's individuality and unique way of coping with labor. She must be able to read her client's moods and respond accordingly.

She must be genuinely enthusiastic about her job. She must be likeable. She must be able to think clearly. She must be tactful. She must have good timing--knowing when to do something and when to be patient, when to say something and when to be silent. She must be a progressive thinker. She must accept change easily. She needs to be resilient; she must have the ability to bounce back after disappointments. She is creative, and often invents new solutions to old problems. She convinces others that these new solutions are worthy and can be used effectively. She considers the feelings of others with whom she works.

Being a labor assistant is complex, yet a very simple role. In the end, assisting women at birth is merely caring for people and helping families to let birth teach them lessons about themselves and about life. It is helping women to discover and draw on their strength, to do their very best, and to be proud of their effort. Through the efforts of the labor assistant, birth can be made safer and more satisfying. These Special Women can help laboring mothers have a birth that truly goes beyond the limits of ordinary experience.

Resources

Write to the following for information on their services:

American Academy of
Husband-Coached Childbirth
(Bradley Method)
PO Box 5224
Sherman Oaks, CA 91413
(800) 423-2397
jayhathaway@bradleybirth.com
www.bradleybirth.com

AWHONN (Association of
Women's Health, Obstetric and
Neonatal Nurses)
2000 L St. NW
Suite 740
Washington, D. C. 20036
(800)673-8499
www.awhonn.org

ALACE (Association of Labor
Assistants & Childbirth
Educators)
P.O. Box 382724
Cambridge, MA 02238-2724
(617)441-2500
e-mail:alacehq@aol.com
http://alacehq.hypermart.net

Birth & Life Bookstore
A Division of Cascade
Healthcare Products
141 Commercial NE
Salem, OR 97301
(800) 443-9942
onecascade@worldnet.att.net
www.1cascade.com/cascade.htm

Birthworks
P.O. Box 2045
Medford, NJ 08055
(888)862-4784
mailroom@birthworks.org
www.birthworks.org

Childbirth Enhancement
Foundation
1004 George Ave.
Rockledge, FL 32955
(407)631-9977
www.cefcares.org

Childbirth & Family Education
287 Whiteface Mountain Dr.
Johnson, VT 05656
(802) 635-2142
e-mail: pollyp@pwshift.com
www.childbirth.org/CFE.html
For information on labor
assistants, labor support, and
training.

Cutting Edge Press
287 Whiteface Mountain Dr.
Johnson, VT 05656
(802) 635-2142
e-mail: pollyp@pwshift.com
www.childbirth.org/CEP.html
Carries books, labor assistant
birth bags and professional
products. Write for a catalog.

Doulas of North America
(DONA)
13513 North Grove Dr.
Alpine, UT 84004
(801)756-7331
FAX 801/763-1847
www.dona.com

La Leche League International
1400 N. Meacham Rd.
Schaumburg, IL 60173-4048
(847)619-7730
Prdept@llli.org
www.lalecheleague.org

ICEA (International Childbirth
Education Association)
P.O. Box 20048
Minneapolis, MN 55420
(800)624-4934
info@icea.org
www.icea.org

Lamaze International, Inc.
1200 19th St. NW
Suite 300
Washington. D.C. 20036
(800) 368-4404
lamaze@sba.dc.com
www.lamaze-childbirth.com

International Cesarean
Awareness Network, Inc.
1304 Kingsdale Ave.
Redondo Beach, CA 90278
(310) 542-6400
(310) 542-5368 FAX
ICANinfo@aol.com
www.efn.org/~djz/birth/add1095/ican.ht
ml

Seattle Midwifery School
2524 16th Avenue South
Room 300
Seattle, WA 98144
(800)747-9433
FAX (206)328-2840
info@seattlemidwifery.org
www.seattlemidwifery.org

Recommended Reading

Most of these reference books may be found in your local library. Many of them may be ordered from Cutting Edge Press. Those are noted with an asterisk. Write or call for a complete listing of books available by mail order as well as shipping charges applicable.

Books
*Active Birth, Janet Balaskas and Arthur Balaskas, Harvard Common Press: Boston, 1992.

Antepartal and Intrapartal Fetal Monitoring: Essentials of Electronic Fetal Monitoring, Michelle Murray, RNC, MSW. NAACOG: Washington, DC, 1988.

*Birth Balls: Use of Physical Therapy Balls in Maternity Care, Perez, P, Cutting Edge Press, Johnson, Vermont, 2000.

*The Birth Partner: Everything You Need to Know to Help a Woman Through Childbirth, Penny Simkin. Harvard Common Press: Boston.

Birth Reborn, Michel Odent. Pantheon Books: NY, 1984.

*Birthing from Within: An Extra-Ordinary Guide to Childbirth Preparation, Pam England & Rob Horowitz, Partera Press, Albuquerque, New Mexico, 1998.

Birthing Normally: A Personal Growth Approach to Childbirth, Gayle H. Peterson. Mindbody Press: Berkeley, CA, 1981.

Childbirth in America: Anthropological Perspectives, , Karen L. Michaelson and contributors. Bergin and Garvey Publishers, Inc.: South Hadley, MA, 1988.

Childbirth Education: Practice, Research and Theory, Francine Nichols and Sharron Humenick. W.B. Saunders Co.:Philadelphia, 1988.

The Complete Book of Pregnancy and Childbirth, Sheila Kitzinger. Alfred A. Knopf: New York, 1989.

*Doula Programs: How to Start and Run a Private and Hospital-Based Program with Success!, Paulina G. Perez and Deaun Thelen, Cutting Edge Press, Johnson, VT, 1998.

*Easing Labor Pain: The Complete Guide to Achieving a More Comfortable and Rewarding Birth, Adrienne B. Lieberman. Harvard Common Press: Boston, MA, 1987.

Episiotomy and the Second Stage of Labor, Sheila Kitzinger and Penny Simkin editors. Pennypress: Seattle, 1984.

*Gentle Birth Choices: A Guide to Making Informed Decisions About Birthing Centers, Birth Attendants, Water Birth, Home Birth and Hospital Birth, Barbara Harper, R.N., Healing Arts Press, Rochester, VT, 1994.

*A Good Birth, A Safe Birth, Diana Korte and Roberta Scaer. Harvard Common Press: Boston.

*Heart and Hands: A Midwife's Guide to Pregnancy & Birth, Elizabeth Davis, Celestial Arts, Berkeley, California, 1997.

*The New Healing Yourself During Pregnancy, Joy Gardner. The Crossing Press: Freedom, CA, 1987.

Home Birth: A Practitioner's Guide to Birth Outside the Hospital, Stanley E. Sagov, Richard I. Feinbloom, Peggy Spindel, and Archie Brodsky. Aspen Systems Corporation: Rockville, MD,1984.

*Mothering the Mother: How a Doula Can Help you Have a Shorter, Easier, and Healthier Birth, Marshall Klaus, M.D.; John H. Kennell M.D.;Phyllis H. Klaus, M.Ed., C.S.W. Addison-Wesley: Reading, MA, 1993.

Nurse-Midwifery, Helen Varney. Blackwell Scientific Publications, Inc.: Boston, 1980.

Oxorn-Foote Human Labor and Birth, H. Oxorn. Appleton-Century- Crofts: New York, 1980.

*Pregnant Feelings: A Workbook for Pregnant Women and Their Partners, Rahima Baldwin and Terra Palmarini. Celestial Arts: Berkley, CA, 1986.

*Silent Knife: Cesarean Prevention and Vaginal Birth After Cesarean, Nancy Wainer Cohen and Lois J. Estner. Bergin & Garvey: South Hadley, MA, 1983.

Some Women's Experiences of Epidurals: A Descriptive Study, Sheila Kitzinger. The National Childbirth Trust: London, England, 1987.

*Special Delivery: The Choices are Yours, Rahima Baldwin. Celestial Arts: Berkeley, CA, 1986.

*Spiritual Midwifery, Revised Edition. Ina May Gaskin. Book Publishing Co.: Summertown, TN, 1980.

*The Labor Progress Handbook, Penny Simkin and Ruth Ancheta, Blackwell Science, Malden, MA, 2000.

*The Nurturing Touch at Birth, Paulina G. Perez, Cutting Edge Press, Johnson, Vermont, 1997.

*The VBAC Companion, Diana Korte, Harvard Come Press, Boston, 1997.

Transformation Through Birth, Claudia Panuthos. Bergin and Garvey Publishers: South Hadley, MA, 1984.

Unnecessary Cesareans--Ways to Avoid Them, Diony Young and Charles Mahan. ICEA: Minneapolis, 1989.

Vaginal Birth After Cesarean Experience, Lynn Baptisti Richards. Bergin and Garvey: South Hadley, MA, 1987.

Women and Health in America, Judith Walzer Leavitt, editor. University of Wisconsin Press: Madison, WI, 1984.

Women's Health, Volume III, Crisis and Illness in Childbearing, Lois Sonstegard, Karren Kowalski, and Betty Jennings. Grune and Stratton, Inc.: Harcourt Brace Jovanovich, New York, 1987.

Articles

"A randomised trial of the effects of monitrice support during labor: mothers' views two to four weeks postpartum," Hodnett ED, Osborn RW, *Birth,* 16:177-183, 1989.

"Are We Overmanaging Second Stage Labor" Charles Mahan and Susan McKay, *Contemporary Obstetrics and Gynecology,* 25:6, p. 91, June 1985.

"Birth Assistant: New Ally for Parents-to-Be, Beth Shearer, *Childbirth Educator,* pp.26-31, Spring 1989.

"Birth Companions: The Key to a Positive Hospital Birth Experience" Lily Fountain Werbos, *Midwifery Today,* 1:5, pp. 24-25, Winter, 1988.

"Can You Make a Difference in Maternity Care?," Perez, P, *Texas Midwifery,* 4(3&4): 16-17, 1987.

A Challenge to Doula," Barbara Hotelling, *ICEA Forum/Sharing,* 1 (1): 15-16, 1985.

"Characteristics Associated with Perineal Condition in an Alternative Birth Center" *Journal of Nurse-Midwifery,* 29:1, p. 29, Jan-Feb., 1984.

"Childbirth Educator and Monitrice: A Winning Combination," Perez, P, *Midwifery Today,* 1(6):35-45, 1998.

"Coaching the Unprepared Parent," Claudia Horowitz, *ICEA Sharing,* 8 (3), 1981.

"Continuous emotional support during labor in a US hospital: a randomized controlled trial," Kennell JH, Klaus MH, McGrath SK, Robertson S, Hinkley C, *JAMA*, 265:2197-2201, 1991.

"Continuous labor support from labor attendant for primiparous women: a meta-analysis," Bemasko, JW, Leybovich, E, Fahs, M, Hatch, Mc, *Obstet Gynecol*, 88(4 Part2):739-44, Oct 1996.

"Commentary: nurses, doulas, and childbirth educators," Gilliland, AL, *J Perinatal Ed*, 7:18-24, 1998.

"Companionship to modify the clinical environment: effects on progress and perceptions of labour, and breastfeeling," Hofmeyr J, Nikodem VC, Wolman WL, Chalmers BE, Kramer T, *Br J Obstet Gynaecol*, 98: 756-764, 1991.

"Counseling the Pregnant Woman: Implications for Birth Outcomes," Michal Morford, *Personnel and Guidance Journal*, June 1984, pp. 619-623.

"A Doula Rises Early" Jillian Van Nostrand, *Mothering*, pp. 64-67, Spring, 1987.

"Effects of continuous intrapartum professional support on childbirth outcomes," Hodnett ED, Osborn RW, *Res Nurs Hlth*, 12:289-297, 1989.

"The Effect of a Supportive Companion on Perinatal Problems, Length of Labor and Mother-infant Reaction" R. Sosa et.al., *New England Journal of Medicine*, 1980, 303: 597-600.

"The Effect of Continuous Epidural Analgesia on Cesarean Section for Dystocia in Nulliparous Women," J.A. Thorp, V.M. Parisi, P.C. Boylan, and D.A. Johnston, *American Journal of Obstetrics and Gynecology*, 162(1989), pp. 670-675.

"The Effect of Continuous Intrapartum Professional Support on Childbirth Outcomes," E.D. Hodrett and R. Osborn, *Research in Nursing and Health*, Dec, 1989, pp. 289-297.

"Effects of providing hospital-based doulas in health maintenance organization hospitals," Gordon NP, Walton D, McAdams E, Derman J, Gallitero G, Garrett L, *Obstet Gynecol*, 93(3):422-426, 1999.

"Effects of psychosocial support during labour and childbirth on breastfeeding, medical interventions, and mothers' well-being in a Mexican public hospital: a randomised clinical trial," Langer A, Campero L, Garcia C, Reynoso S, *Br J Obstet Gyneacol*, 105: 1056-1063, 1998.

"Effects of social support during partution on maternal and infant morbidity," Klaus MH, Kennell MH, Roberston S, Sosa R, *Br Med J*, 293:585-587, 19 86.

"Epidural Analgesia and Cesarean Section for Dystocia: Risk Factors in Nulliparous Women," J.A. Thorp, Linda Eckert, M.S., D.A. Johnson, and A.M. Peaceman, V.M. Parisi, *American Journal of Perinatology,* vol. 8:6, Nov. 1991, pp. 402-440.

"Induction of labor: an integrated review, " Bramadat, IJ, *Health Women Int*, 15(2):135-48, Apr 1994.

"Induction of labor and doula support," McGrath SK, Kennell JH, *Pediatric Res* 43(4):Part II, 14A, 1998.

"Journeying through labour and delivery: perceptions of women who have given birth, " Leaphart, WL, Meyer, MC, Capeless, EL, *J Maternal Fetal Med*, 6(2):99-102, Mar-Apr 1997.

"Just Another Day in a Woman's Life? Women's Long-Term Perceptions of Their First Birth Experiences." Simkin, P, *Birth*, 18(4):203-210, 1991.

"Labor Support by a doula for middle-income couples during labor; the effect on cesarean rates," Kennell, JH, McGrath SK, *Pediatric Res*, 32:12A, 1993.

"Labor Support in Relation to Birth Outcomes," Adrienne Bennett et.al., *Birth*, Spring, 1985, vol. 12., no. 1., pp. 9-15.

"Labor Support Makes it a Labor of Love, Barbara Hotelling, *ICEA Forum/Sharing*, 1(1): 15-16, 1985.

"Lessons from Home Birth," *Childbirth Educator*, Summer 1988, pp. 34-38.

"Let Your Couples Know about the Role of the Professional Labor Assistant," Perez, P, *IJCE*, 4(2):39, May 1989.

"Massage for Childbirth" Mirka Knaster, *East-West Journal*, July 1985, pp. 57-62.

"The Midwife as Doula: A Guide to Mothering the Mother," Dana Raphael, *The Journal of Nurse Midwifery*, 26 (6), pp. 13-15, 1981.

"Mothering the New Mother" Johnetta Frick Rodrigues, *MS Magazine*, May 1986.

"My Way: The Support of a Third Person During Labor Helps an Expectant Couple Enormously" Beth Shearer, *Childbirth Educator*.

"Natural childbirth: nurses in private practice as monitrices." Hommel F, *Amer J of Nursing*, 69:1446-50, 1969.

"Nurses: work sampling study in an intrapartum unit, " Gagnon, AJ, Waghom, K, *Birth*, 23(1):1-6, Mar 1996.

"Nursing support of the laboring woman," Hodnett, E, J *Obstetecol Neonatal Nurs*, 25(3):257-64, Mar-Apr 1996.

"Nurturer of Laboring Women in a High Tech Town, " Perez, *Childbirth Alternative Quarterly*, 3: 1985.

"Position in Labour: A Plea for Flexibility,CNelki J, Bond L, *Mod Midwife*, 5(2):19-22, Feb 1995.

"Postpartum depression and companionship in the clinical birth environment: a randomized, controlled study," Wolman WL, Chalmers B, Hofmeyr J, Nikodem VC, *Am J Obstet Gynecol*, 168:1399-1393, 1993.

"The Changing Role of the Labor Partner," Deborah Regal, *ICEA Sharing*, XI:2:84, pp. 3,11.

"The effects of doula support during labor on mother-infant interaction at 2 months," Martin S, Landry S, Steelman, Kennell JH, McGrath, S, *Infant Behav Develop*, 21: 556, 1998.

"The effects of doula support during labor on mother-infant interaction at 2 months," Landry SH, McGrath, SK, Kennell JH, Martin S, Steelman L, *Pediatric Res*, 43(4):Part II, 13A, 1998.

"The effects on whirlpool baths in labour: a randomized, controlled trial, " Rush, J. Lambert, K, Loosley-Millan, M, Hutchison, B, Enkin, M, *Birth*, 23(3):136-143, Sep 1996.

"The effect of a supportive companion on perinatal problems, length of labor, and mother-infant interaction." Sosa R, Kennell H, Klaus MH, Roberston S, Urrutia, *N Engl J Med*, 303:597-60, 1980.

"The Patient Observer: What Really Happened at the Bedside?" Perez, P., *Birth*, 15(3):171-178, Sep 1998.

"The Patient Observer: What Really Led to these Cesarean Births?" Perez, P, *Birth*, 16(3):130-139, Sept 1989.

"The Obstetrical and Postpartum Benefits of Continuous Support during Childbirth," Scott KD, et al, *J of Women's Health & Gender-Based Medicine*, 8(10): 1257-1264, 1999.

"The Return of the Doula," Barbara Hotelling, *Genesis*, Aug.-Sept. 1986, vol. 8, no. 4, pp. 9,10,12.

"Satisfaction with care in labor and birth: a survey of 790 Australian women," Brown, S, Lumley, J, *Birth*, 21(1):4-13, Mar 1994.

"Should We Fire the Coach?," *Childbirth Educator*, 1988.

"Social support during premature labor: effects on labor and the newborn," Cogan R, Spinnato JA, *J Pyschoson Obstet Gynaecol*, 8:209-216, 1988.

"Someone to Watch Over Her," Paulina Perez, *Childbirth Instructor,* Autumn 1993, pp. 22-26.

"Support During Labor Good Common Sense" R. Cogan, *ICEA Review*, April, 1984, Vol. 8, No. 1.

"Ways and knowing about birth in three cultures," Sargent, C, Bascope, G, *Modn Anthropol Q*, 10(2):213-26, June 1996.

"Why Hire Labor Support" Marilyn Lucey, *C/SEC Newsletter*, p. 1- 2, April, 1985.

"Women's perceptions of nursing support during labor," Bryanton, J, Fraser-Daveym H, Sullivan, P, *Obstet Gynecol Neonatal Nursing*, 23(8):638-44, Oct 1994.

A Seminar for Doulas

Paulina Perez is available to conduct learning seminars for those interested in becoming a doula. Besides being the author of *Special Women: The Role of the Professional Labor Assistant*, the first book on the topic of professional labor support, Ms. Perez is an internationally known perinatal nurse and lecture. Her expertise is gleaned from years of experience and has enabled her to keep her finger on the pulse of current changes in health care. Her energetic speaking style and her ability to make complex information easily understandable make her a much sought after speaker.

This seminar is designed to help participants become expert labor assistants. Lecture, discussion, slides, videos, and experiential learning sessions are part of the course curriculum. Topics covered include: emotions and psychological processes of labor and birth, comfort measures, prenatal and postpartum discussion topics, ethics and standards, referral sources, communication skills, and values clarification. In this seminar, Ms. Perez draws on her experience attending over 600 births as a professional labor assistant to address issues that are important to labor support providers. The two day course will fulfill partial requirements needed for certification with Doulas of North America (DONA).

Call (802) 635-2142, write her at C.F.E., Inc., 287 Whiteface Mountain Dr., Johnson, VT 05656, or check her website at www.childbirth.org/CFE.html for detailed information about holding a seminar for doulas in your area as well as for current schedule of Ms. Perez' speaking engagements. Send email to pollyp@pwshift.com.